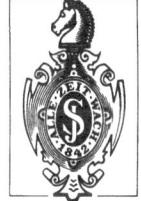

P. Regazzoni Th. Rüedi R. Winquist
M. Allgöwer

The Dynamic Hip Screw
Implant System

With 45 Figures in 119 Separate Illustrations

Springer-Verlag
Berlin Heidelberg New York Tokyo 1985

PD Dr. *Pietro Regazzoni*
Departement Chirurgie der Universität, CH-4031 Basel

Prof. Dr. *Martin Allgöwer*
Hebelstrasse 2, CH-4031 Basel

Prof. Dr. *Thomas Rüedi*
Departement Chirurgie, Rätisches Kantonsspital Chur,
CH-7000 Chur

Robert Winquist, M.D.
Orthopedic Physicians, Inc., P.S., Suite 1600,
901 Boren Avenue, Seattle, WA 98104/USA

ISBN-13:978-3-642-69927-6   e-ISBN-13:978-3-642-69925-2
DOI: 10.1007/978-3-642-69925-2

Library of Congress Cataloging in Publication Data. Main entry under title:
The Dynamic hip screw implant system. Bibliography: p. Includes index. 1. Hip
joint-Fractures-Treatment. 2. Bone screws (Orthopedics). 3. Internal fixation in
fractures. I. Regazzoni, P. (Pietro), 1944–. II. Title: Hip screw implant system.
(DNLM: 1. Bone Screws. 2. Fracture Fixation, Internal. 3. Hip Fractures-sur-
gery. WE 855 D997)   RD549.D96   1985   617′.581044   84-13998

© Springer-Verlag Berlin Heidelberg 1985
Softcover reprint of the hardcover 1st edition 1985

2124/3140-543210

Contents

1 Introduction

The AO/ASIF* dynamic hip screw (DHS) has been designed primarily to stabilize trochanteric fractures of the hip. Selected fractures of the femoral neck and some subtrochanteric fractures are further indications for the DHS [40, 46]. The dynamic condylar screw (DCS) has been developed for fractures of the distal femur and is now being tested clinically. The DHS and DCS are carefully coordinated with the preexisting ASIF standard sets of equipment for internal fixation of fractures.

The concept of a sliding screw for trochanteric fractures is not new. The first author describing such an implant was Schumpelick [44]; he gives credit to Pohl [22], who was primarily a manufacturer working for Gerhardt Künscher. He described the possibility of impaction at the fracture site with a sliding device. In the United States Clawson [7, 8] introduced the hip screw and found it to be extremely beneficial in trochanteric fractures. At approximately the same time, Massie [31, 32] and Pugh [39] designed the sliding-type flange nails, which offer similar intramedullary splinting with the possibility of fracture impaction.

The following chapters describe the concept and design features of the DHS, as well as the details of the surgical technique. The application of the DHS for different types of fractures is illustrated with clinical examples. The results of 268 cases of trochanteric fractures treated with the DHS are presented and compared with results using the angled blade plate and Ender's nails. Finally, some laboratory tests are described.

---

* AO, Arbeitsgemeinschaft für Osteosynthesefragen; ASIF, Association for the Study of Internal Fixation

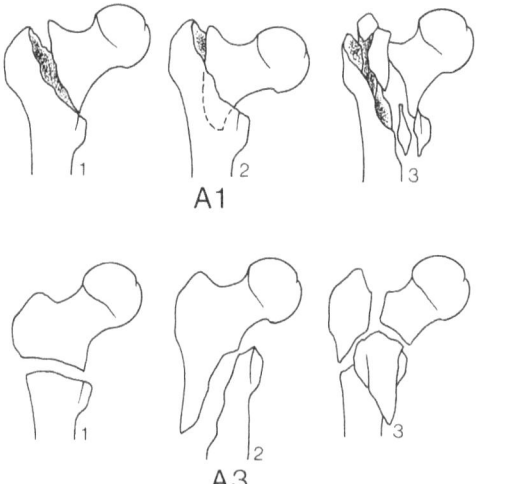

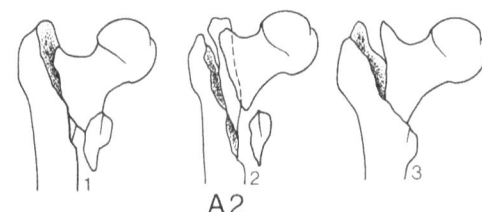

Fig. 1. ASIF classification of trochanteric fractures. *A1,* single; *A2,* multiple; *A3,* intertrochanteric

In the absence of solid bony support of the opposite cortex (i.e., without valgization) the cyclic bending (varus) forces and torsional stresses are transmitted to the fixed-angle nonsliding device. If the fracture is not consolidated within 2–3 months, one or more of the following complications are likely to occur:

1. Breakage of implant at the blade-(nail)-plate junction due to metal fatigue
2. Blade penetration into the acetabulum, or actual cutout of the blade
3. Pullout or breakage of screws in the lateral cortex of the femur

With intramedullary devices such as Ender's nails, the weight bearing stress – in case of unstable fractures (loss of posteromedial buttress) – will very often cause the collapse of the femoral neck and a varus deformation, with distal migration of the nails or nail penetration into the acetabulum.

In contrast, the DHS allows not only stable fixation of anatomically reduced trochanteric fractures but also a guided collapse and impaction of the fragments in the unstable fracture. The screw will slide distally and laterally until a new area of bony support is reached. The implant will therefore not be unduly stressed (load-sharing instead of load-bearing device) and the fracture will usually unite. Some shortening will result, but significant functional disabilities due to this are rare. By this "impaction" the complications mentioned – especially implant failure due to metal fatigue – and nail migration are prevented in most instances.

2 The Problem of Trochanteric Fractures

Trochanteric fractures generally occur in elderly patients. The average age of patients is about 75 years. Women (70%) are more than twice as often concerned as men.

Comminuted fractures are frequent because of the osteoporosis typical for this age group. Preexisting medical problems (cardiovascular disease, severe central nervous system disfunction, chronic respiratory disease, and diabetes) are regularly found. In these patients the main goal is *early mobilization* in order to avoid the complications of prolonged bed rest. Early ambulation, however, nearly always means full weight bearing, since the elderly patient is seldom able to walk with partial weight bearing [30, 34, 40, 42].

The aim of open reduction and internal fixation of trochanteric fractures is therefore to obtain optimal functional results in all types of trochanteric fractures with a *low complication rate,* by means of a *short operation* which should *not be too demanding technically*.

Classification

According to the ASIF classification [33] (Fig. 1), three groups of trochanteric fractures can be distinguished, depending on whether the medial cortex shows an intact lesser trochanter, i.e., a single or several fractures, or fractures of both cortices. The ASIF classification allows a differentiated comparison of the results of different series of trochanteric fractures and the distinction between stable (type A1) and unstable (most of type A2 and A3) trochanteric fractures.

Problems in Fixation

The treatment of stable trochanteric fractures usually presents very few hazards and will be successful with any type of implant, provided it is applied in the proper way [25].

In unstable fractures, however (particularly types A2.2, A2.3, and A3.3), complications are frequent [10, 15, 18, 19, 40] if a fixed-angle, nonsliding implant is used. The application of angled blade plates in unstable fractures must usually be combined with a valgus osteotomy and medial displacement of the femoral shaft in order to prevent fatigue of the plate [10, 20, 34]. This means a technically very demanding operation and extensive exposure of the fracture site with an increased infection rate. Furthermore, functional results are not very satisfying.

3 DHS Implant System

Design Features

The DHS implant system is composed of the DHS plate and the DHS lag screw. The plates are available with two types of barrels: a standard barrel (38 mm) and a short barrel (25 mm). The short barrel plates are seldom indicated; their gliding characteristics are far less satisfactory than those of the standard barrel plate. Their use should be limited to especially small femurs and to the rare cases where a long impaction distance is to be expected and where the screw might "run out of glide" with a standard barrel. In cases where medial displacement osteotomy is carried out, the use of the short barrel might be advisable.

The DHS plates are produced with several barrel angles (135°, 140°, 145°, 150°), but in the great majority of cases a 135° plate is best. It must be realized that the technical problems of correct placement of the implant increase with greater plate angles, although greater angles may offer biomechanical advantages (better gliding characteristics, reduction of bending stresses on tube-plate junction), particularly in unstable cases. A wide selection of plate lengths (2, 4, 5, 6, 8, 10, and 12 holes) for the 135° (and the 150°) plates helps the surgeon in adapting to various fracture situations. The 140° and 145° plates exist in only three lengths (4, 5, and 6 holes). Lag screws are available from 50 mm up to 145 mm in length, in 5-mm increments.

Standard Surgical Technique

Trochanteric Fracture – 135° DHS

The operation is performed with the patient in a supine position, and we prefer the use of a regular operating table. The patient may be placed on a fracture table, although this takes more time and to us seems rather a disadvantage, particularly for the comminuted fracture types, because it may render reduction quite difficult.

One image intensifier is indispensable and allows for axial as well as AP viewing; some authors, however, prefer two image intensifiers.

The extremity is draped freely in order to facilitate manipulation of the leg. Using traction, abduction, and internal rotation, and sometimes slight flexion about the knee, even very severely dislocated and comminuted fractures can be reduced. Without the fracture table a temporary fixation of the reduced fragments with one or two Steinmann pins is advisable. The results of the reduction manoeuvers can be checked by means of the image intensifier.

Exposure

The proximal femur is exposed by means of a straight lateral incision on the thigh, beginning at the greater trochanter and running toward the lateral femoral condyle, the length depending on the size of the DHS plate chosen. The fascia lata is split in the same direction. The origin of the vastus lateralis is incised in its posterior half and along the linea aspera. The proximal femur is now exposed by reflecting the vastus anteriorly. Any perforating vessel must be identified and ligated. Usually no further exposure of the fracture is required.

To determine the anteversion of the femoral neck a solid Kirschner wire is slid over the front of the femoral neck, using the appropriate angle guide with the T-handle, and hammered slightly into the head (Fig. 2).

The point of introduction of the guide pin is determined preoperatively on the X-ray of the fracture. The level varies with the angle of the plate to be used. In the great majority of cases, when a 135° plate is used the guide pin is introduced at a point approximately 2.5 cm below the tuberculum innominatum (the rough line of the greater trochanter). The lesser trochanter can also be used as a landmark. The middle of the lesser trochanter would usually be the entry point for a 135° plate. The angle guide is placed against the middle of the femoral shaft with the guide tube pointing to the center of the femoral head. The lateral cortex is opened with a 2-mm drill (optional). The DHS guide pin is inserted in the center of the femoral head to the level of subchondral bone. *The pin must remain in place throughout the procedure.* The threaded end of the guide pin helps to prevent accidental backing out (Fig. 3).

If the guide pin is inadvertently withdrawn it must be reinserted. A correct repositioning is possible using the short centering sleeve and a DHS lag screw inserted backward in the centering sleeve as guides (Figs. 4, 5). If the guide pin is not correctly reinserted there is a considerable risk of placing the lag screw in a wrong direction, away from the original bore hole, especially in porotic bone [11].

The exact placement of the guide pin into the center of the femoral head is the most important step of the surgical procedure. If the guide pin lies correctly and the operative technique is followed as described, major technical problems are unlikely to occur during the rest of the procedure.

The guide pin must lie in the middle of the femoral neck; its position must therefore be checked radiographically in both AP and axial views (Figs. 6, 7). If a fracture table is used the axial X-ray is somewhat impractical to take. Without the fracture table the axial view may be obtained by a 90° flexion, 30° abduction, and slight external rotation of the hip, with the image intensifier pointing in the AP direction (Fig. 7). (In these cases the fracture must of course be secured by one or two Steinmann pins placed cranialy to the future DHS position. To minimize the risk of fracture dislocation during this manipulation traction should be exerted on the thigh).

The tip of the guide pin must lie just short of the joint space to allow the correct measurement. If the pin position is not perfect it must be changed before any further step is taken.

To measure the length of the inserted guide pin the DHS "direct measuring device" is slipped onto the guide pin and the length of pin inserted into the proximal femur is read directly (Fig. 8, e.g., 105 mm). The frontal Kirschner wire may now be removed.

As the drill hole should end 10 mm short of the joint surface, we subtract 10 mm from the reading and set the reamer to the correct depth, (e.g., $105-10=95$ mm; Fig. 9). The DHS triple reamer provides three functions in one operation: reaming for the lag screw, the barrel, and the plate-barrel junction. The depth of the reamer is adjustable in 5-mm increments.

When the different portions of the reamer enter the lateral cortex, the pressure exerted on the reamer should be diminished in order to avoid further damage to the bone. This is particularly important when the entry point is close to the fracture.

For extremely hard cancellous bone – as encountered in young patients – the threads for the lag screw should be precut with a DHS tap, using the shorter of the two centering sleeves (Fig. 10).

Figure 11 gives an example of measurements:
1. Measurement 105 mm
2. Reamer setting: 95 mm
3. Tap (optional): 95 mm
4. Lag screw length: 95 mm

In *osteoporotic* bone the screw is inserted as far as the 5-mm mark (the lag screw cutting itself the last 5-mm of the thread). In hard bone the screw is inserted as far as the 0-mm mark on the wrench.

The following instruments mentioned are illustrated in Fig. 12: Insert DHS coupling screw (1) into hollow DHS guide shaft (2), screw male thread (1) into female thread of lag screw (3); the ridge and slot between the guide shaft and the lag screw must interdigitate (4). Slide the longer of the two centering sleeves over the DHS wrench (5). Glide the DHS wrench over the guide shaft-lag screw assembly and slip the centering sleeve over the guide pin into the bore hole (see Fig. 13). Insert the lag screw by turning the handle clockwise and exerting a gentle push.

If too much force is needed to introduce the screw, it may be safer to check the position of the device with the imageintensifer, or to back out and use the tap first.

The lag screw is inserted until the 0 mark on the DHS wrench reaches the lateral cortex. This means that the lag screw is 10 mm from the joint line. In osteopoenic bone the screw may be inserted about 5 mm deeper (see Figs. 11 and 14).

The handle of the wrench must be placed parallel to the shaft of femur, before it is removed together with the centering sleeve.

After removal of the wrench, the appropriate DHS plate is slid onto the assembly (Fig. 15). The coupling screw is loosened and the guide shaft and guide pin are removed.

The plate should be gently seated with the impactor (Fig. 16). The DHS plate is fixed to the femur with 4.5-mm ASIF cortex screws. The DCP neutral drill guide, 3.2-mm drill bit, and standard AO/ASIF techniques should be used for screw insertion (Fig. 17).

A final impaction of the fracture can be achieved with a DHS compression screw (Fig. 18); however, this is rarely indicated. In osteoporotic bone the compression screw must be tightened carefully to avoid stripping the thread of the DHS lag screw. Manual impaction of the fragments after the side plate has been attached to the shaft and impaction by early weight bearing are probably much more effective than impaction with a compression screw. Removal of the compression screw is optional (Fig. 19).

Additional subtrochanteric fragments can be fixed by means of lag screws, through the plate or independent to it (Fig. 20).

Wound Closure and Postoperative Management

The placement of one or two suction drains below the fascia lata is recommended. The fascia is closed with resorbable suture material (Vicryl or Dexon).

We do not advocate the routine use of prophylactic antibiotics, as their efficacy is still a matter of controversy [5]. There is, however, a selected group of high-risk patients who should receive antibiotics for 24–48 h. In every patient some sort of prophylaxis against thromboembolism (low-dose heparin, coumarin, or Dextran 70) is advocated, starting preoperatively or soon after the operation.

The patients are encouraged to get out of bed early, if possible the day after surgery. For aged people this usually means full weight bearing, which either has to be accepted or taken into consideration. There is no doubt that the rehabilitation process is facilitated by allowing the elderly to use both legs for ambulation.

Implant Removal

First remove the DHS plate. Then put the DHS wrench over the lag screw and insert and fix the long coupling screw into the female thread of the lag screw. Turn the wrench counterclockwise, pulling on it at the same time (Fig. 21).

In patients over 70 years of age the implant is usually not removed. However, formation of a painful bursa or local pain over a migrated implant due to collapse of the femoral neck might indicate plate removal. In younger people the implants are always removed after about 1 year.

Particular Technical Problems

Femoral Neck Fractures

Although the DHS was designed and is advocated mainly for fractures in the pertrochanteric to subtrochanteric area, it may also be used in lateral fractures of the femoral neck.

The fractures should be reduced in a slight valgus overcorrection. An extra Steinmann pin, placed parallel and well proximal to the central guide pin (Fig. 22), holds the reduction and prevents the femoral head from rotating during reaming, taping, and screw insertion. After removal of the Steinmann pin it may be replaced by a 6.5-mm cancellous bone screw to additionally lock rotation.

Unstable Trochanteric Fractures with Posteromedial Comminution

In these fractures care must be taken to avoid a posterior angulation of the proximal fragment, as the posteromedial buttress is missing. As there is a certain danger of placing the guide pin eccentrically into the rather weak anterosuperior quadrant, it is essential to check the pin position very carefully on the image intensifier in the axial projection (the entire femoral head and neck must be shown on the TV screen). The guide pin must lie in the middle of the neck and head in both planes (Fig. 23), even if there is no bony contact in the postero-medial comminuted area. To prevent rotation of the femoral head these unstable fractures may also be secured with an additional Steinmann pin (see Femoral Neck).

Four-Part Fractures

As in femoral neck fractures, in the so-called four-part fracture a stabilizing Steinmann pin is necessary to avoid rotating of the proximal fragment while reaming and inserting the lag screw (Fig. 24).

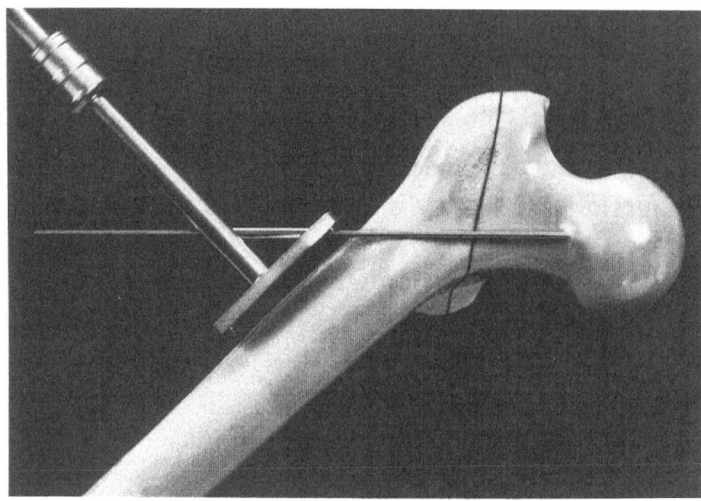

Fig. 2. Determination of axis of femoral neck

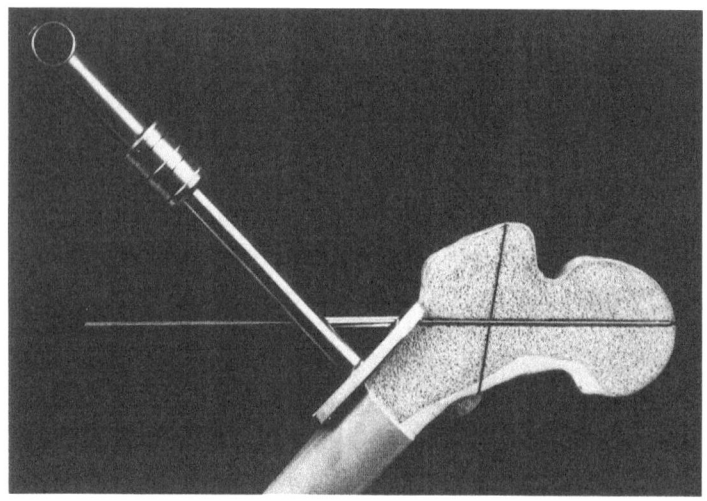

Fig. 3. Placement of guide pin

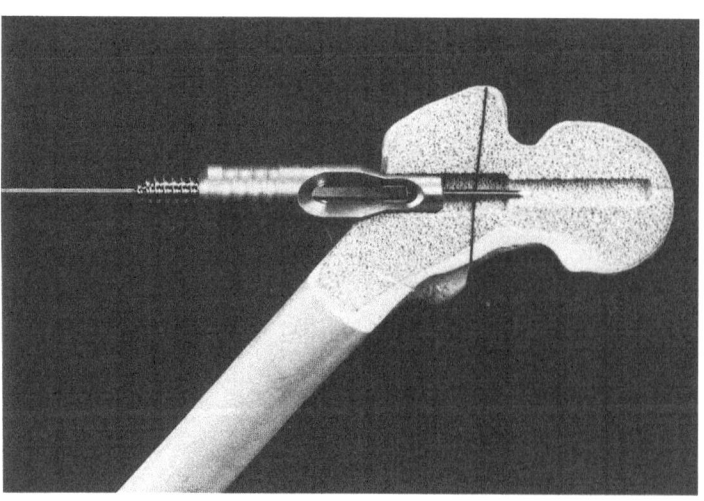

Fig. 4. Reinsertion of guide pin after inadvertent withdrawal

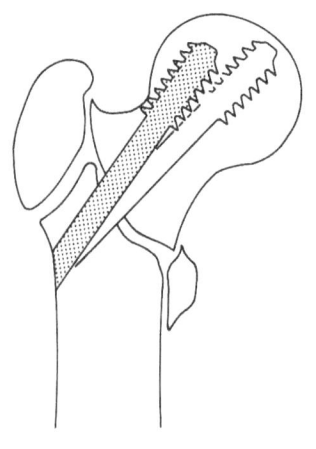
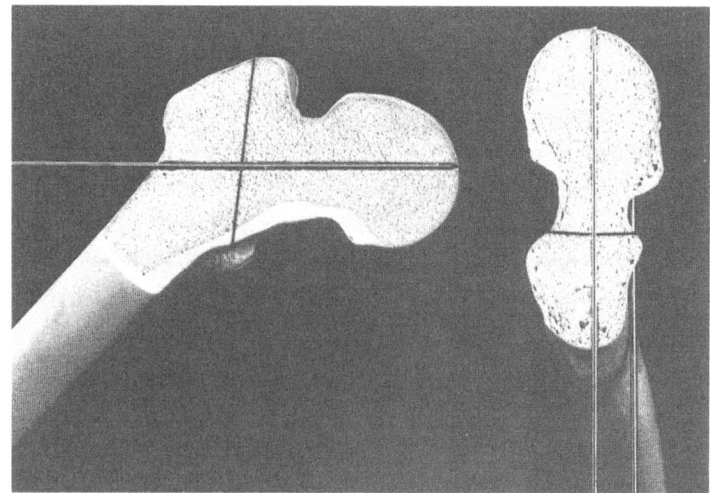

Fig. 5 (left). Incorrect position of lag screw inserted without guide pin in place

Fig. 6 (right). Correct position of guide pin (AP and axial view)

Fig. 7. Position of leg for radiographic control: axial view

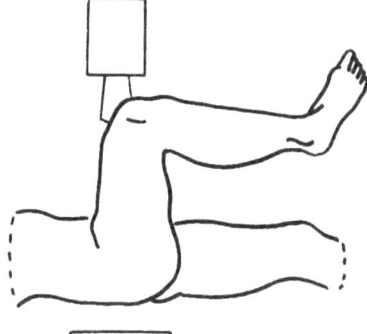
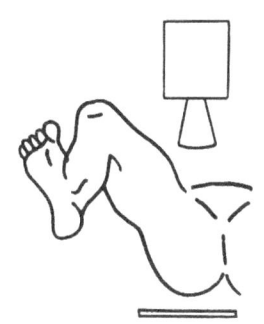

Fig. 8. Direct measuring of guide pin length

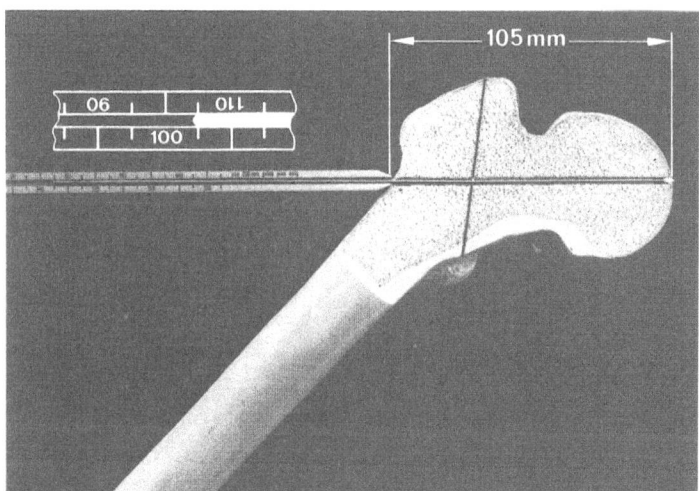

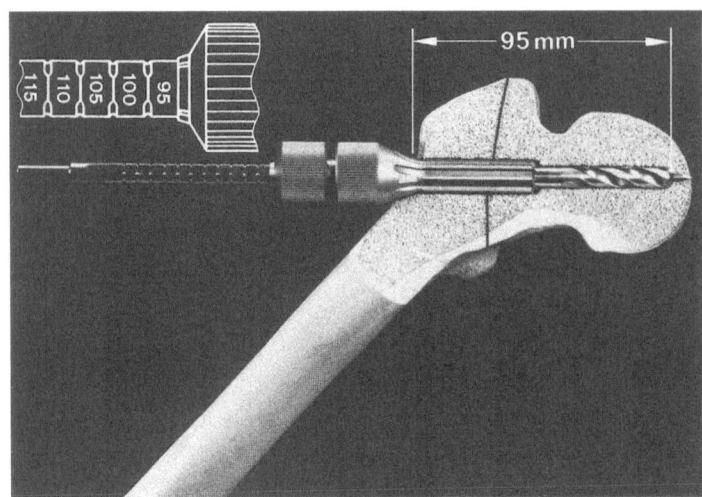

Fig. 9. Reaming with triple reamer

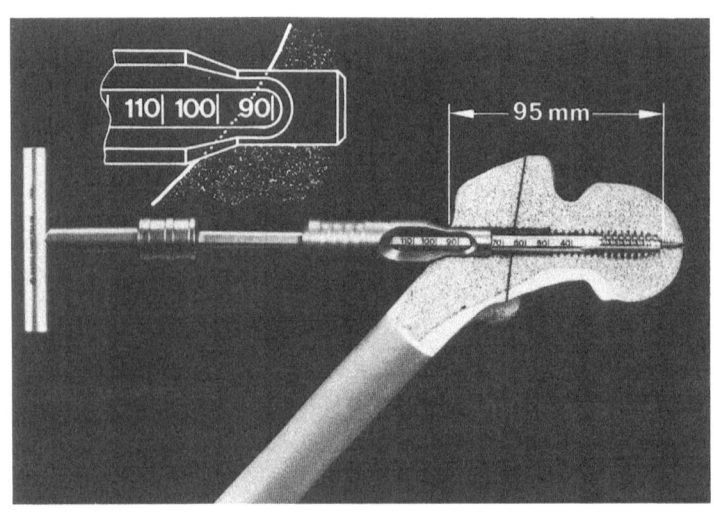

Fig. 10. Taping

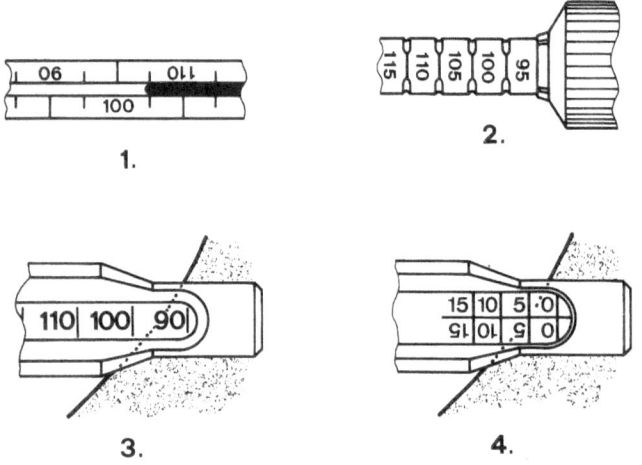

Fig. 11. Practical example

1. Direct measurement (105 mm)
2. Setting of triple reamer (105 − 10 = 95)
3. Taping as far as 95 mm
4. Introduction of DHS-screw at −5, which allows for some compression

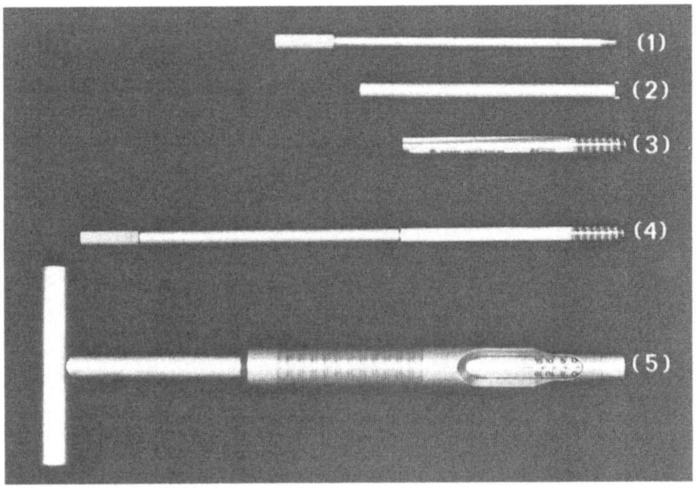

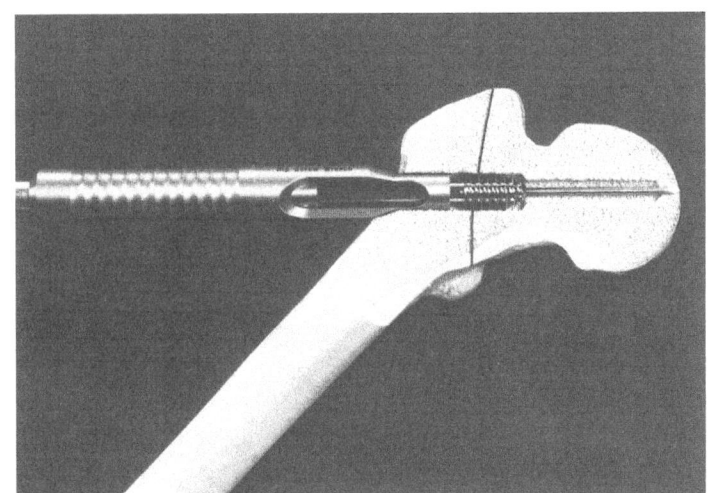

Fig. 12. Introduction of lag screw 1: single elements

(1) Coupling screw
(2) Guide shaft
(3) DHS-screw
(4) Assembly of 1–3
(5) DHS-wrench with long centering sleeve

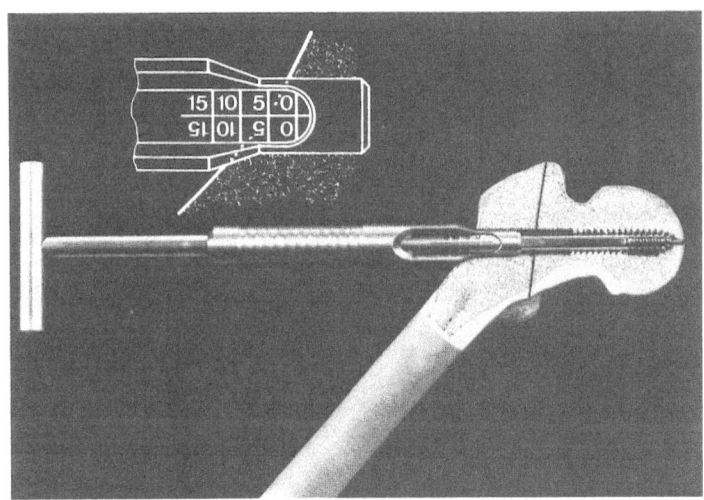

Fig. 13. Introduction of lag screw 2: single elements assembled

Fig. 14. Introduction of lag screw 3: final position

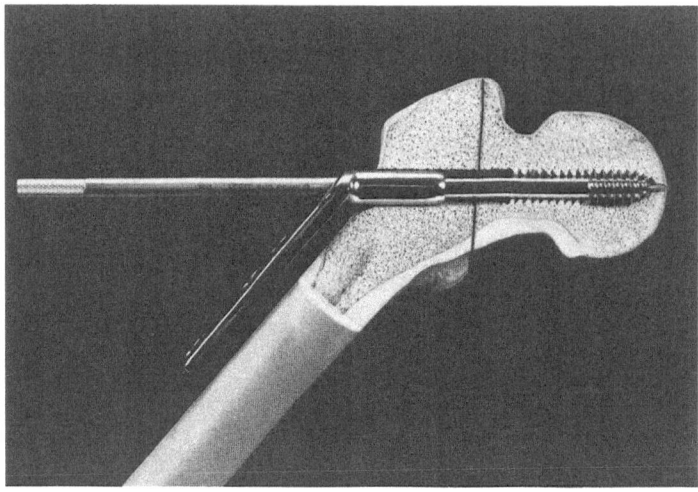

Fig. 15. Placement of DHS plate

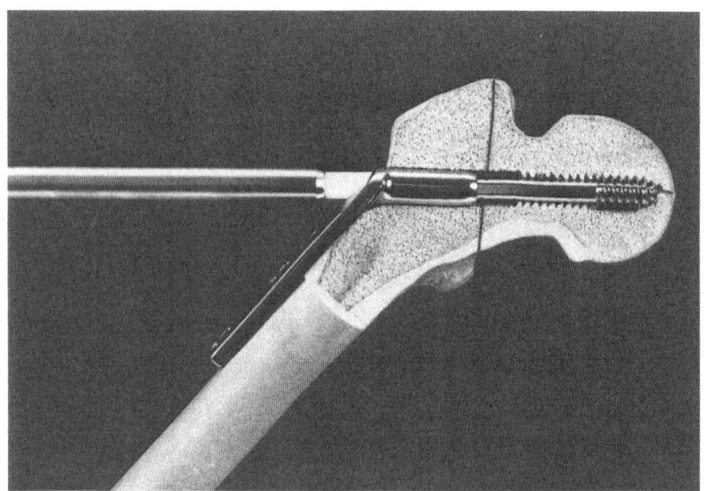

Fig. 16. Impaction

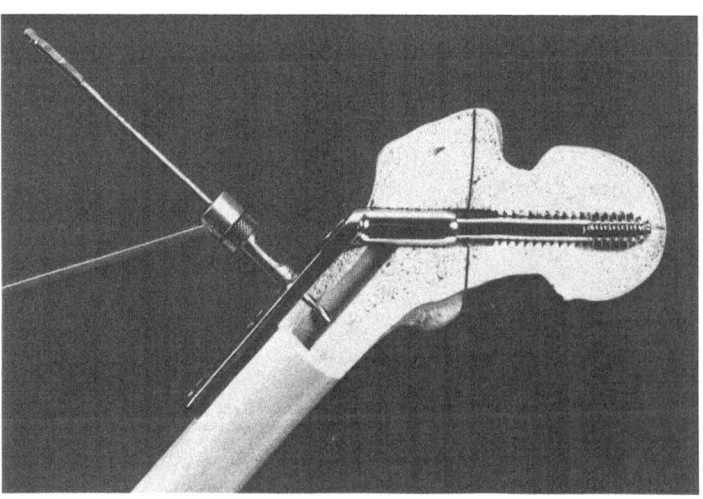

Fig. 17. Plate fixation

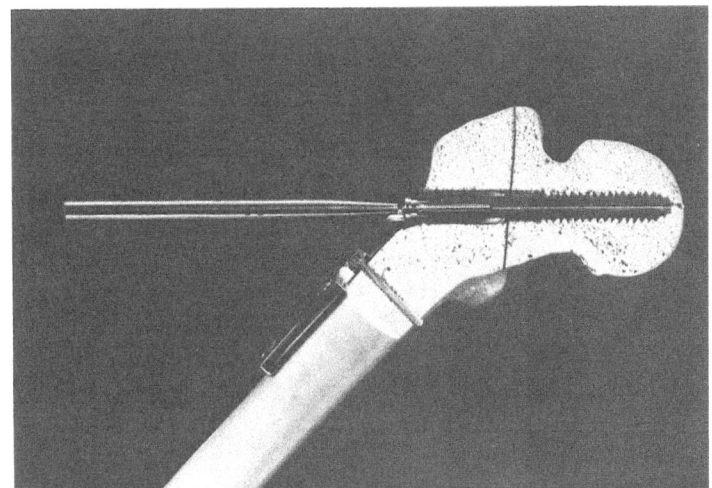

Fig. 18. Final impaction with DHS compression screw

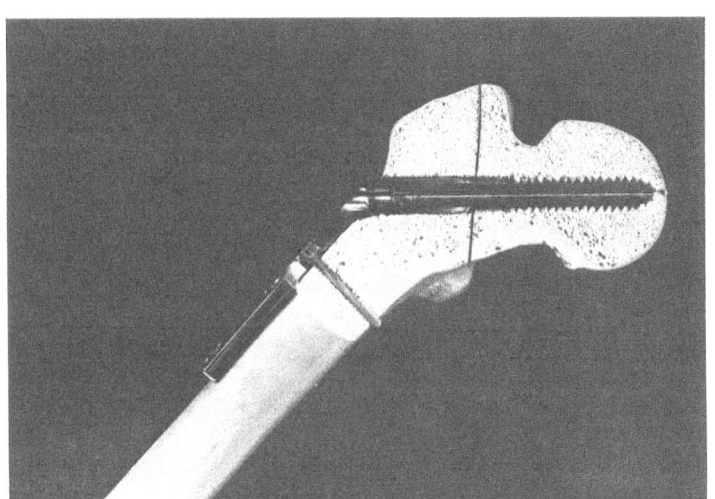

Fig. 19. Removal of compression screw

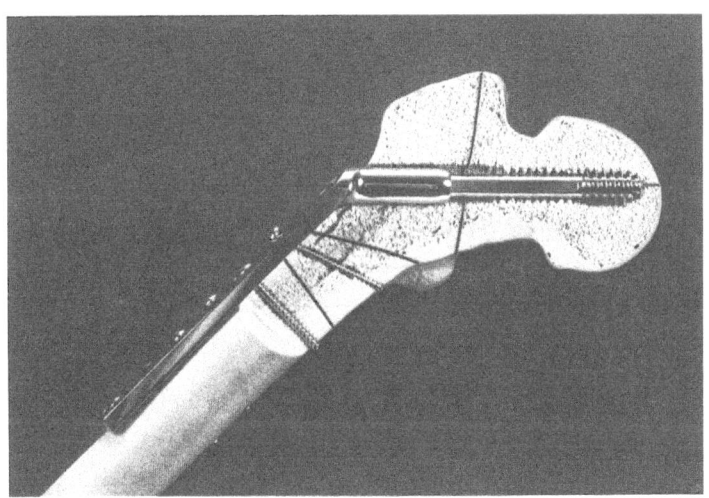

Fig. 20. Fixation of subtrochanteric fragments

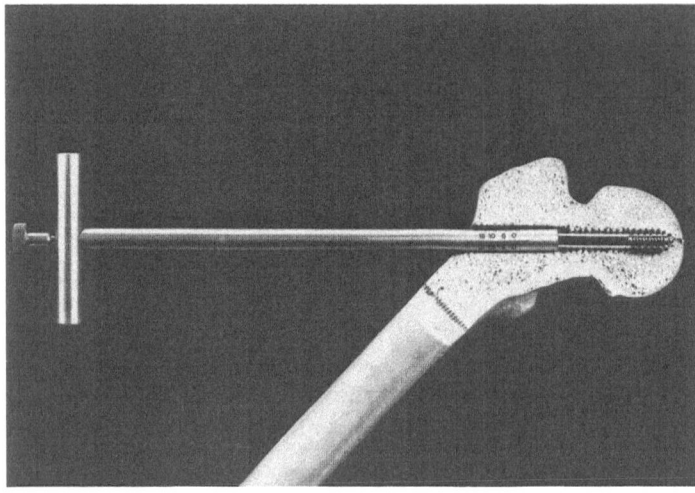

Fig. 21. Implant removal

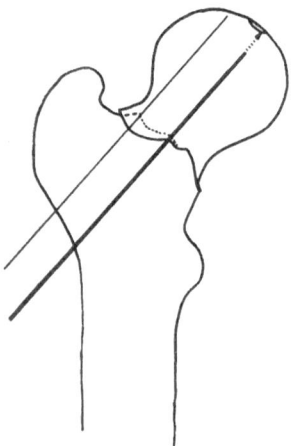

Fig. 22. Femoral neck fracture: preliminary fixation with Steinmann pin, placement of guide pin

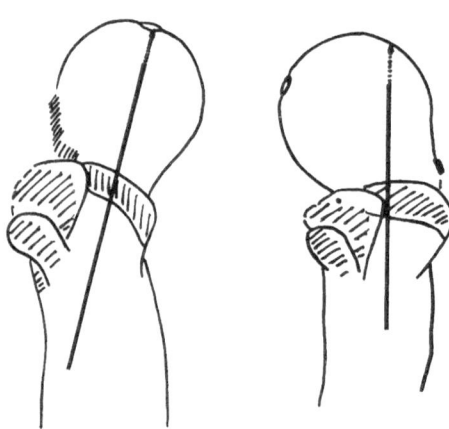

Fig. 23. Trochanteric fracture with comminution. *Left:* correct reduction and guide pin placement; *right:* posterior angulation of proximal fragment, incorrect anterior placement of guide pin

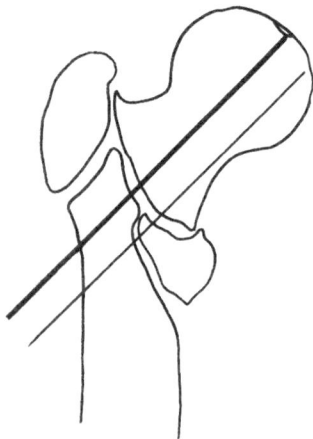

◁*Fig. 24.* Four-part fracture: preliminary fixation with Steinmann pin

4 Application of the DHS: Clinical Examples

The indication for operative treatment of hip fractures is universally accepted. However, there is a great deal of controversy about what is the best implant for internal fixation. For example, with neck fractures, some surgeons advocate primary prosthetic replacement rather than internal fixation. In trochanteric fractures, Ender's nails, angled blade plates, and various types of gliding hip screws are the implants most frequently proposed.

Following a series of examples of the clinical use of the DHS (Figs. 25–38), a comparison of Ender's nails, angled blade plates, and the DHS for trochanteric fractures illustrates our clinical experience of the past 10 years.

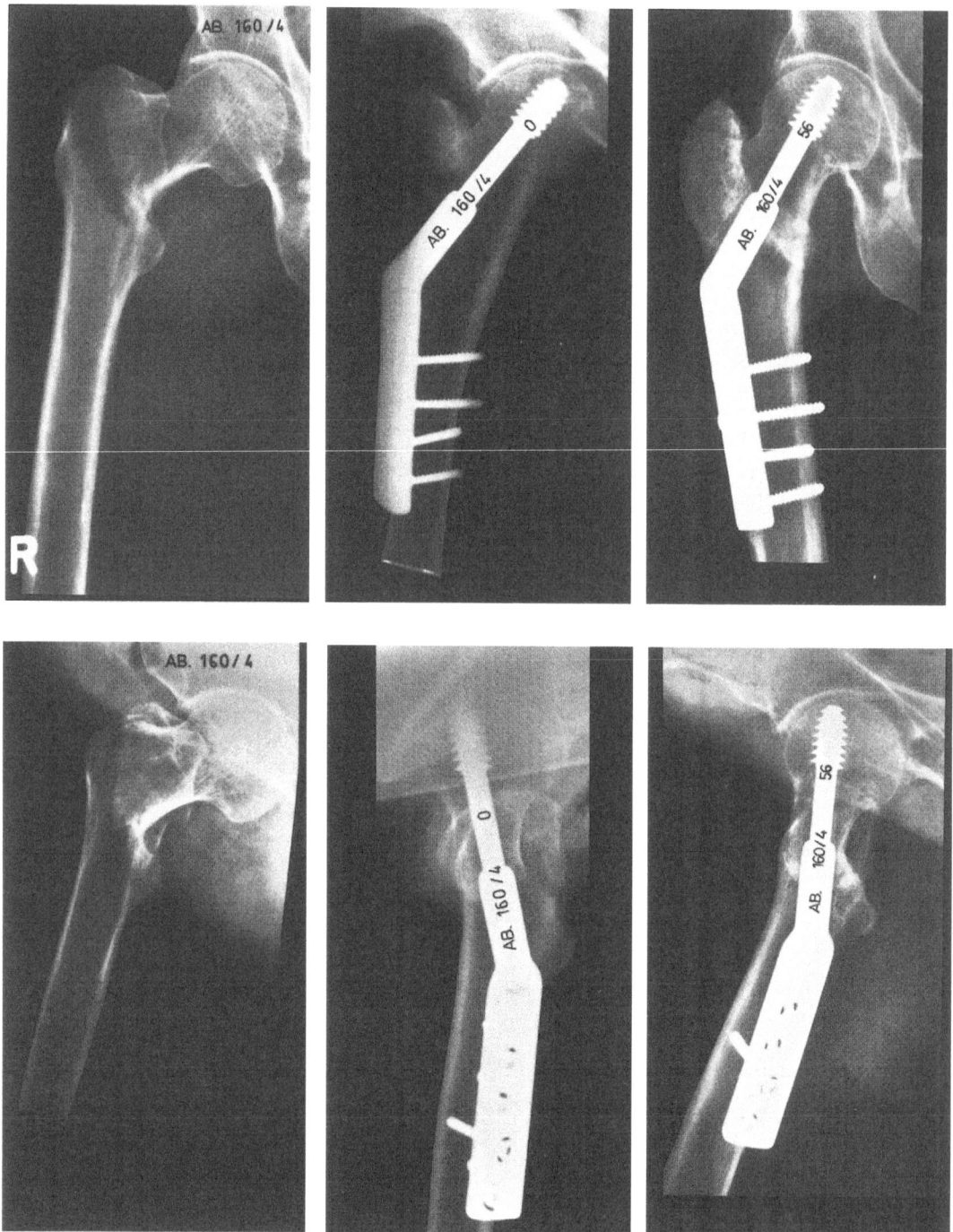

Fig. 25. Stable trochanteric fracture, type A.1.1, in a 73-year-old woman. Fixation with 135° DHS. Immediate full weight bearing; uneventful healing; good functional result

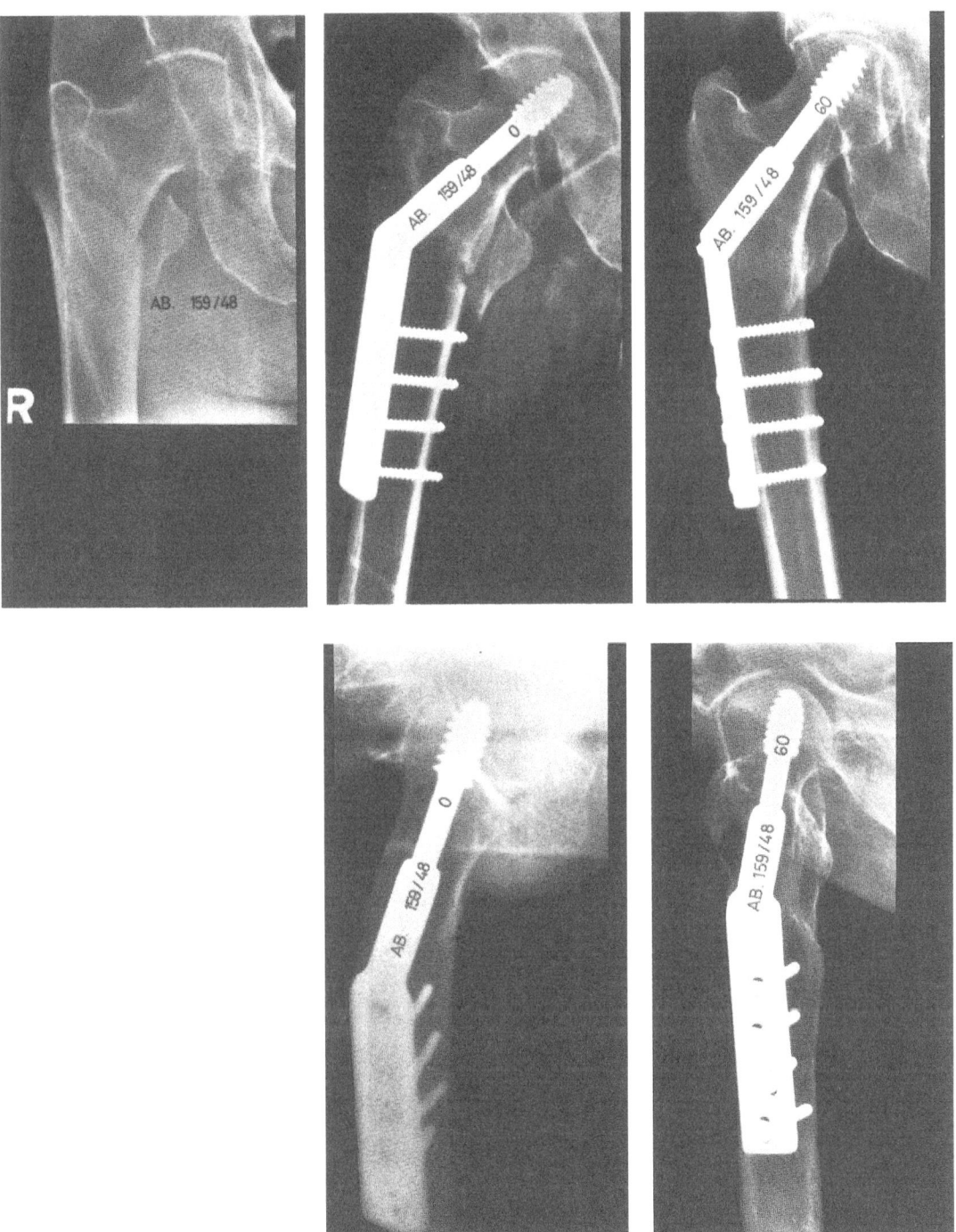

Fig. 26. Fracture, type A.2.2, in a 76-year-old woman. 135° DHS fixation and uneventful healing. Note that no attempt was made to fix the lesser trochanter

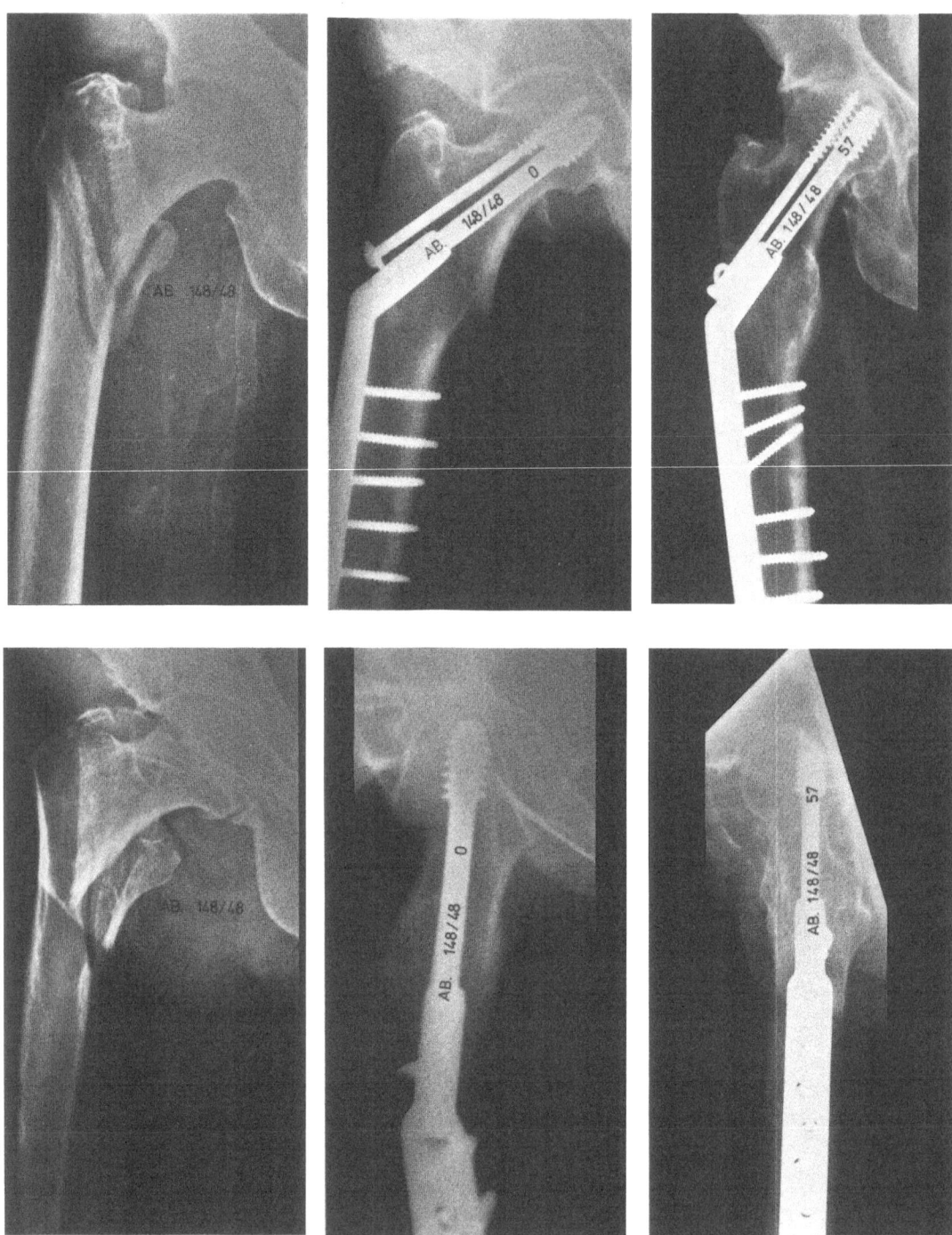

Fig. 27. Type A.2.3 fracture in a 76-year-old woman. Fixation with DHS and additional lag screw. Healing is uneventful, however, *any* additional screw in the femoral neck and head should be avoided, if not parallel, as it might impede an effective gliding process

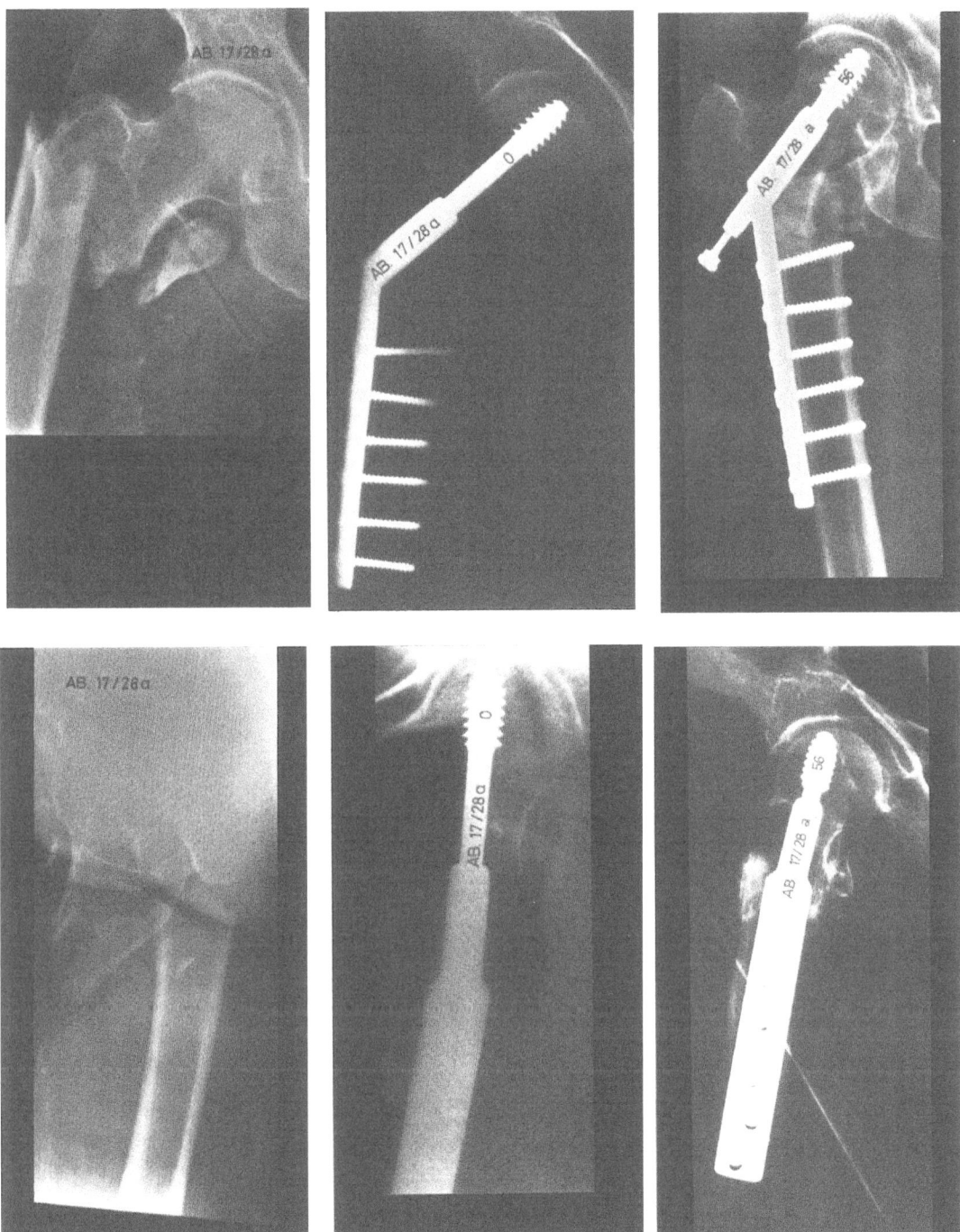

Fig. 28. Intertrochanteric fracture, type A.3.1, in an 83-year-old woman. Fixation with 135° DHS and six-hole plate. Because of severe osteoporosis a longer plate than usual was chosen. Important telescoping. The compression screw used in this case was not necessary (cf. Fig. 12); fortunately, there was no discomfort due to the protruding lag screw and compression screw. Uneventful healing

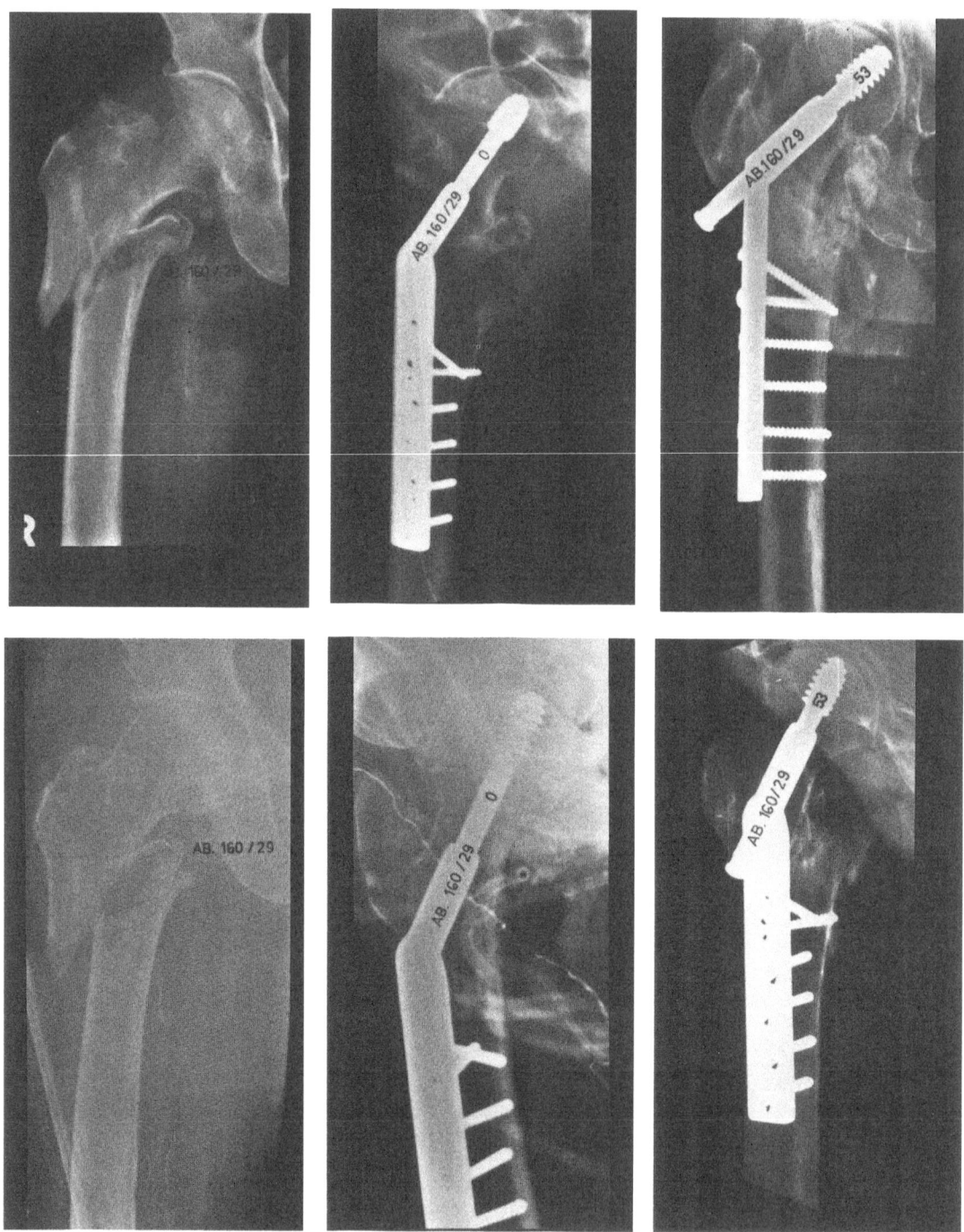

Fig. 29. Unstable intertrochanteric fracture, type A.3.2, in a 72-year-old woman. Reduction and 135° DHS fixation. Immediate full weight bearing; important telescoping; uneventful bone union. Leg shortening of 2 cm; good range of movement

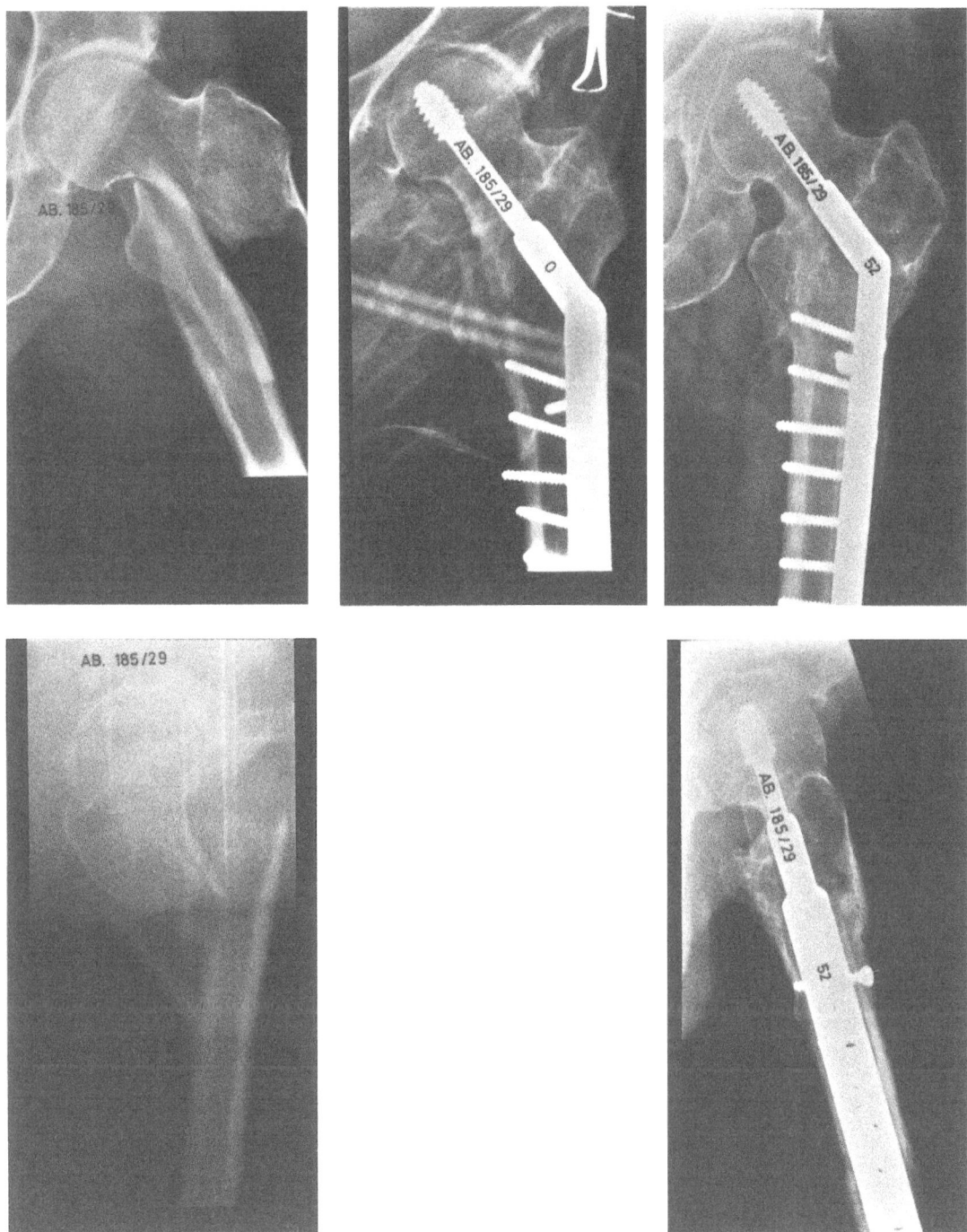

Fig. 30. Combined trochanteric and subtrochanteric fracture, type A.3.3, in a 55-year-old man (classification according to the fracture level presenting the greater technical problems). 135° DHS, eight-hole side plate, three lag screws through the plate, additional lag screw outside the plate

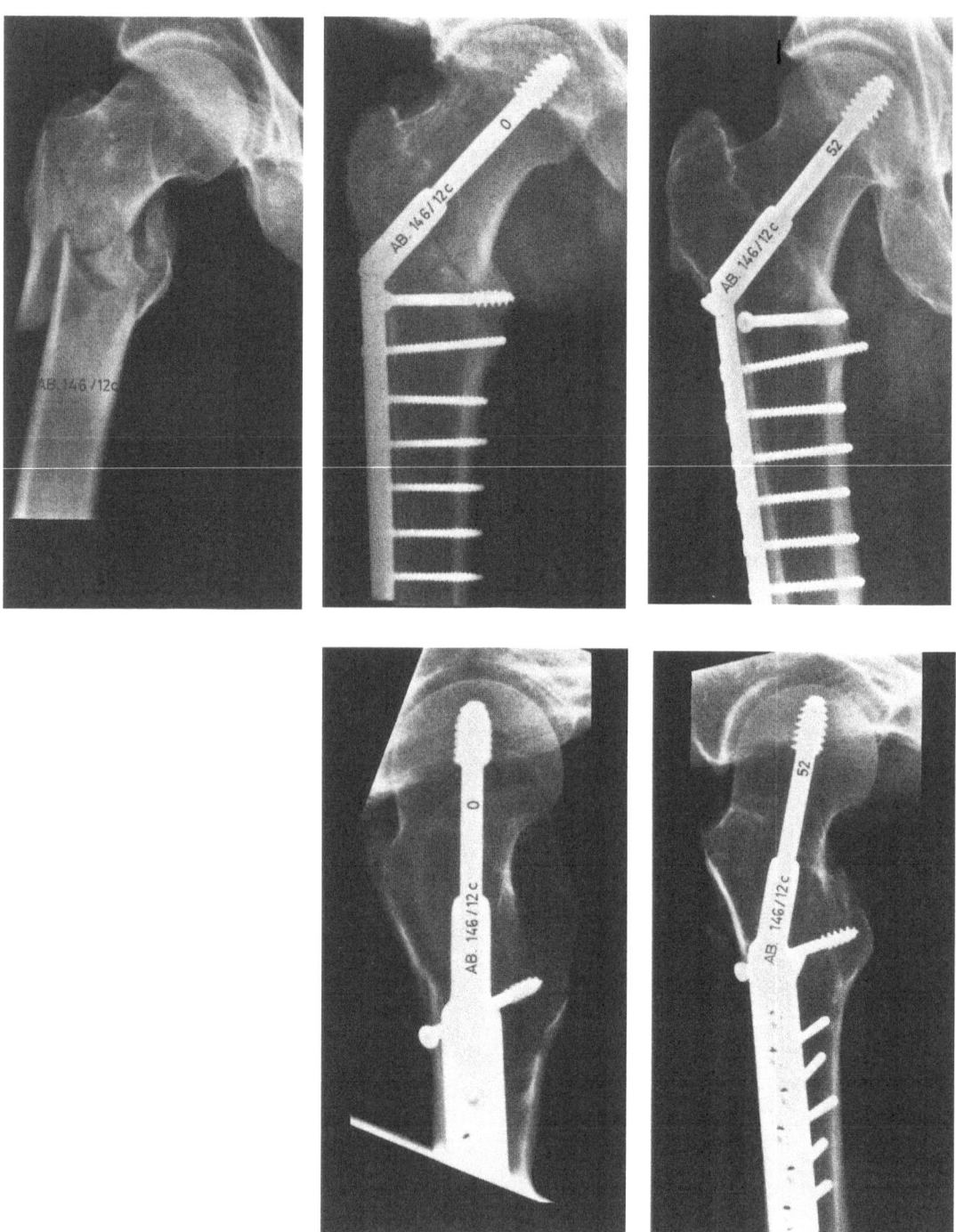

Fig. 31. Unstable intertrochanteric fracture, type A.3.3, in a 52-year-old man. Anatomical reduction and fixation with 135° DHS and additional lag screw for the lesser trochanter. Partial weight bearing for 8 weaks; uneventful bony union; full range of movement. X-rays show result at 52 weeks

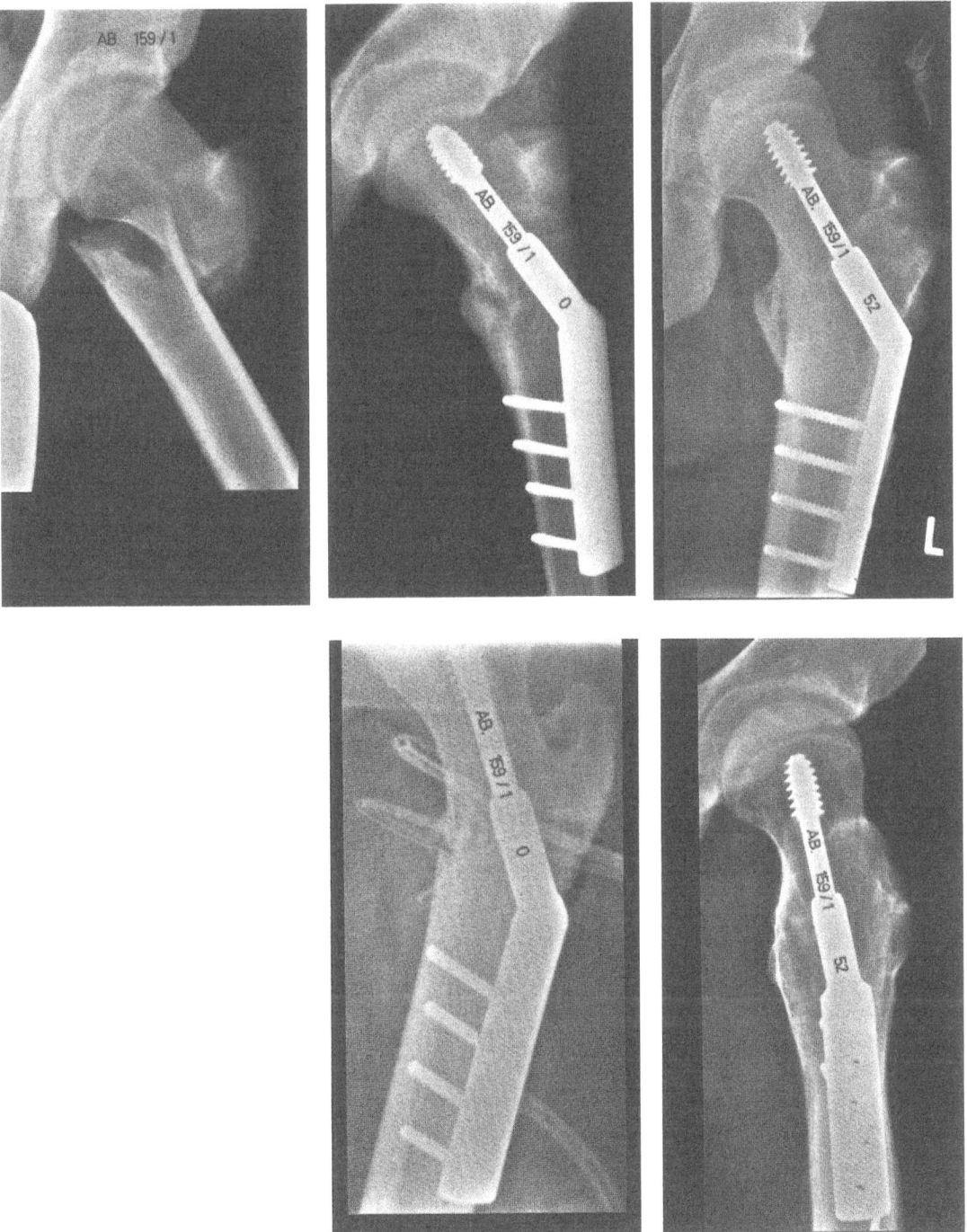

Fig. 32. Trochanteric fracture, type A.3.1, in a young man of 16 years with an open epiphysis. Fixation with DHS. Uneventful healing; X-rays show result after 52 weeks. Full range of movement

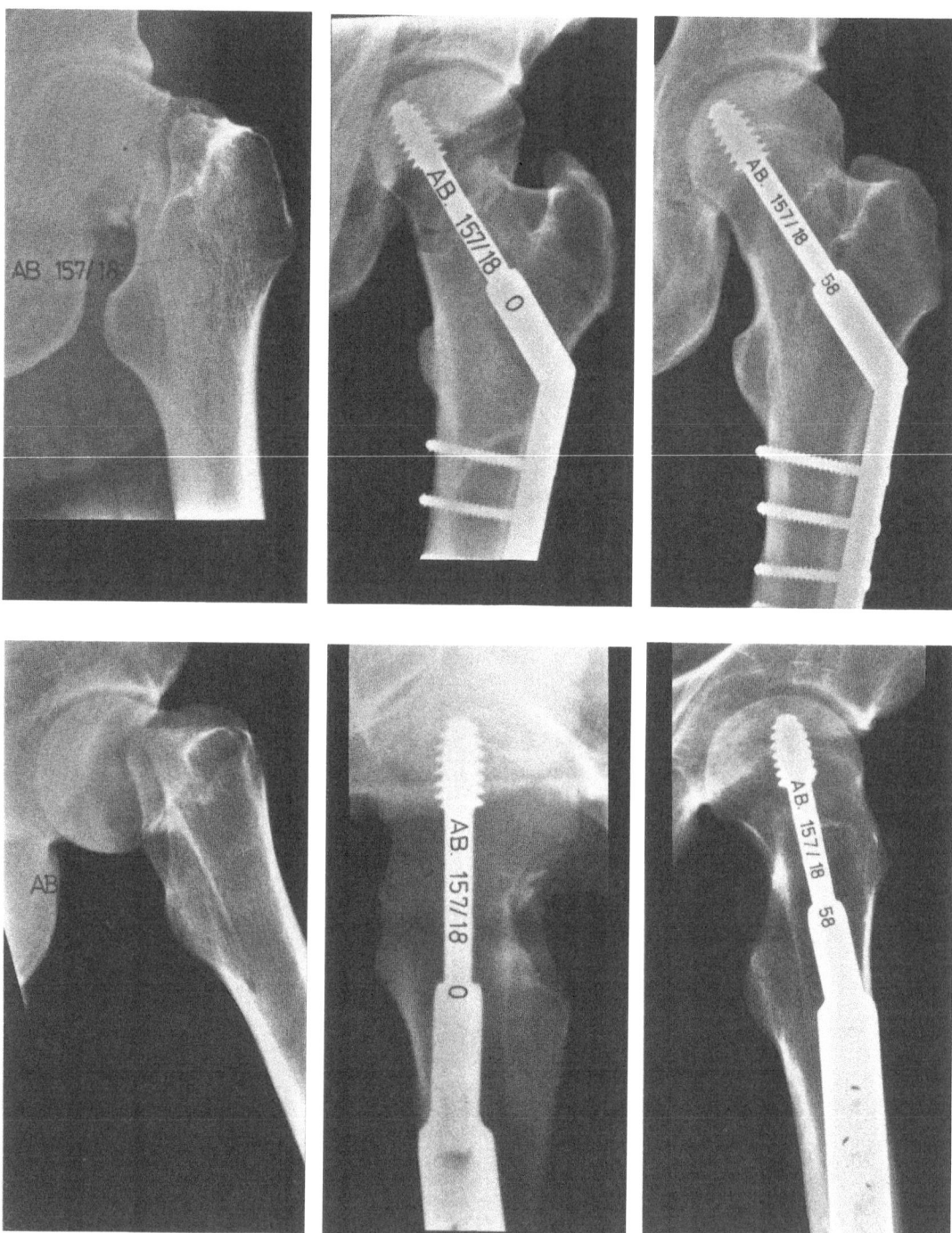

Fig. 33. Femoral neck fracture in a 28-year-old man. Reduction with slight valgus overcorrection. Fixation with four-hole DHS plate; a two-hole plate would have been sufficient. Partial weight bearing for 3 months. No signs of avascular necrosis of the head after 58 weeks

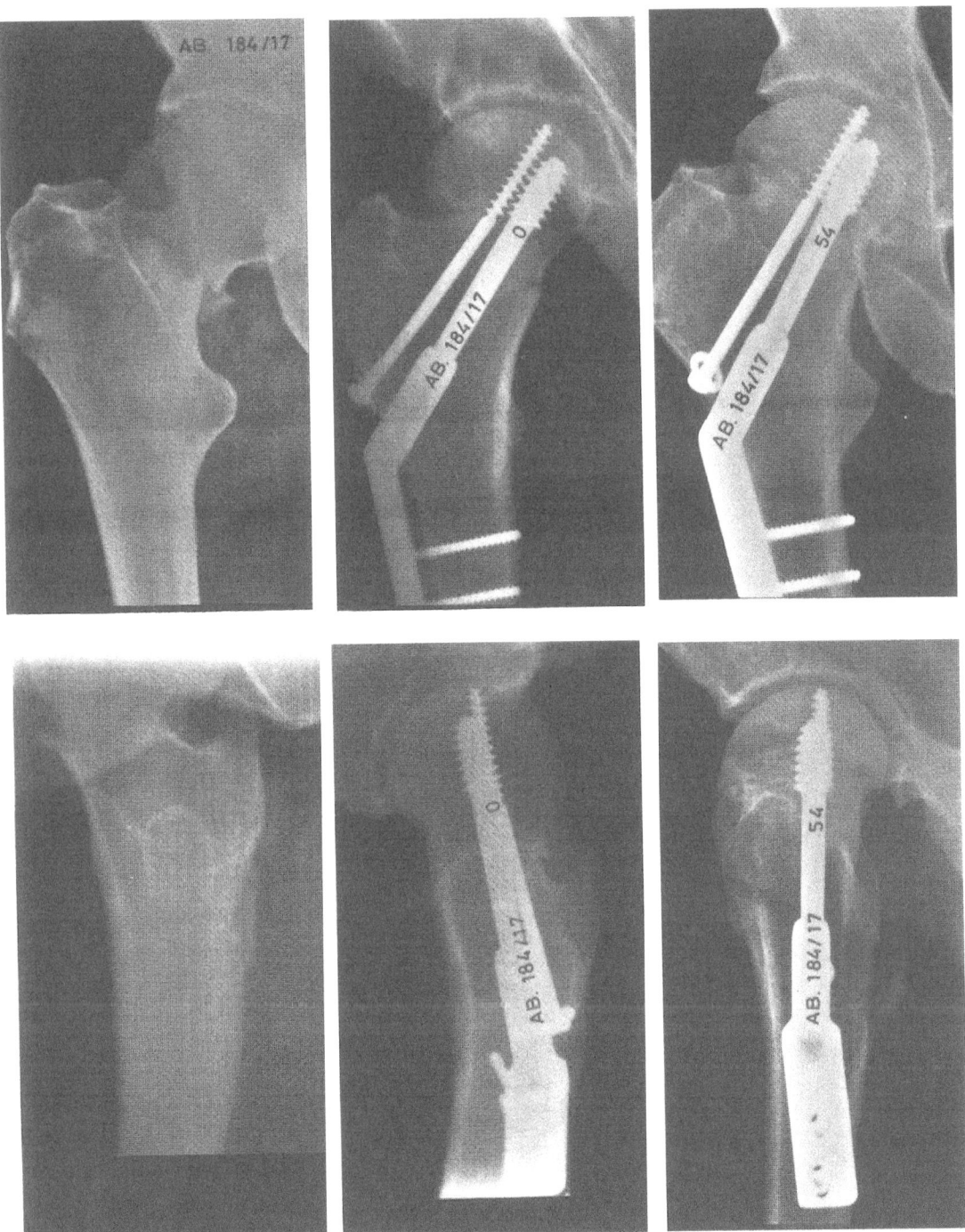

Fig. 34. Femoral neck fracture in a 54-year-old man. Reduction with valgus overcorrection and stabilization with 135° DHS. The additional lag screw used here is not necessary, and might have impeded impaction if it were not strictly parallel to the DHS

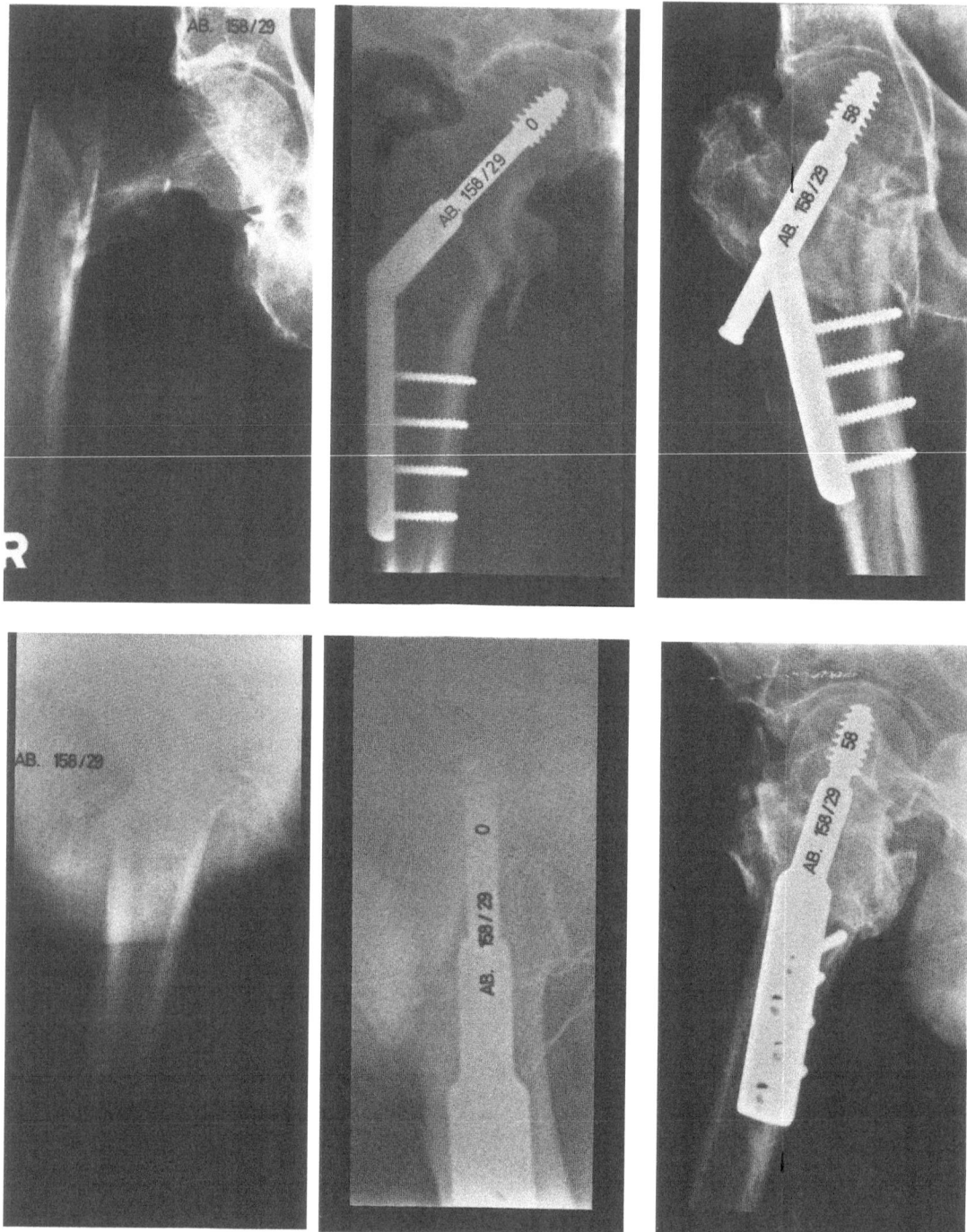

Fig. 35. Unstable trochanteric fracture, type A.2.3, in an 82-year-old woman. Fixation with DHS. Immediate full weight bearing. Impaction of the fracture until a new bony buttress is found; considerable telescoping. Fracture healed with shortening of the leg by 2 cm. Only slight local discomfort at the site of the protruding screw; implant removal refused

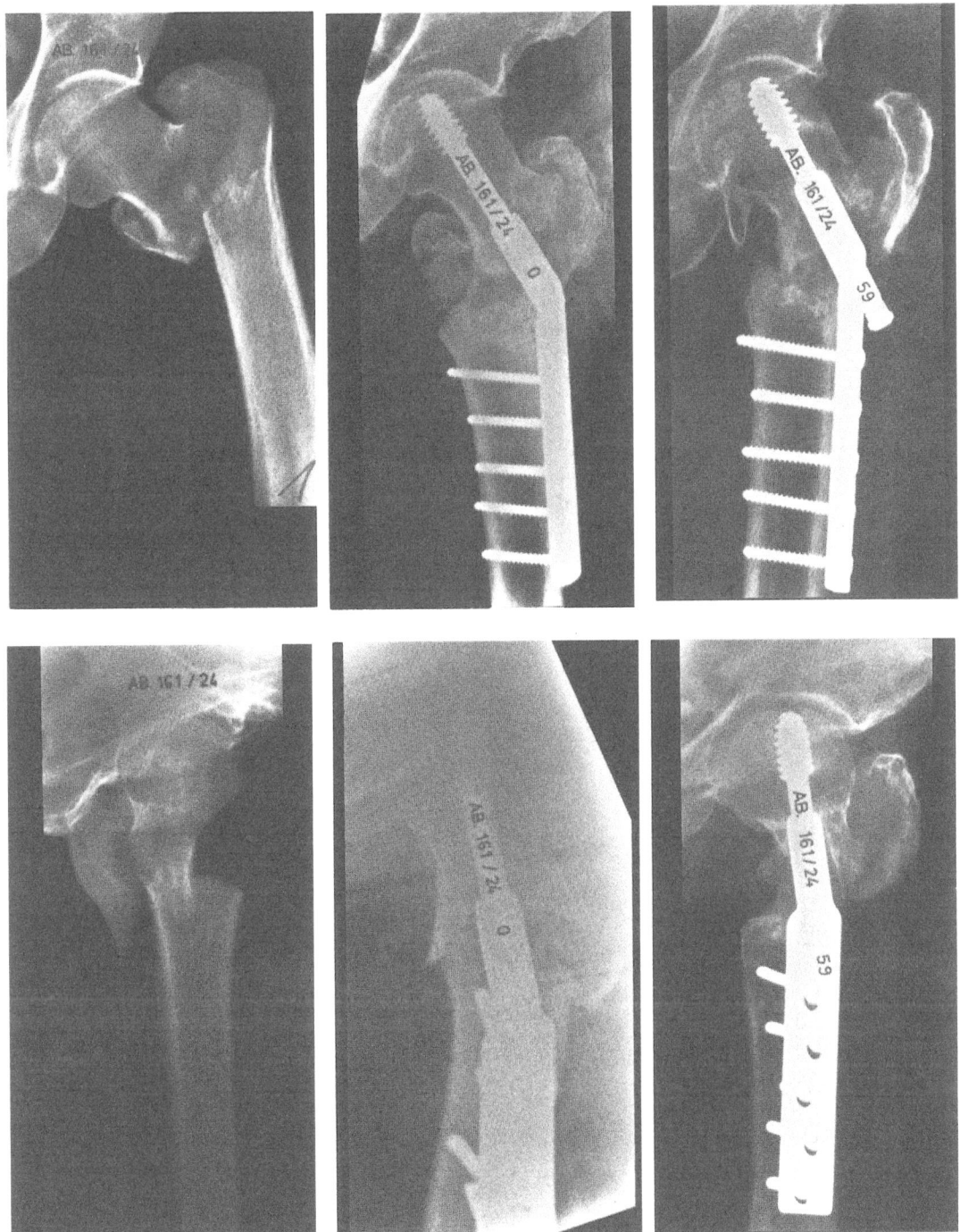

Fig. 36. Type A.2.3 fracture in an 85-year-old woman. The 145° DHS is a "forgiving" implant-healing occurred despite poor reduction and bad screw placement. No tension band wire for the greater trochanter was used. Patient walking with 1.5-cm shortening of left leg

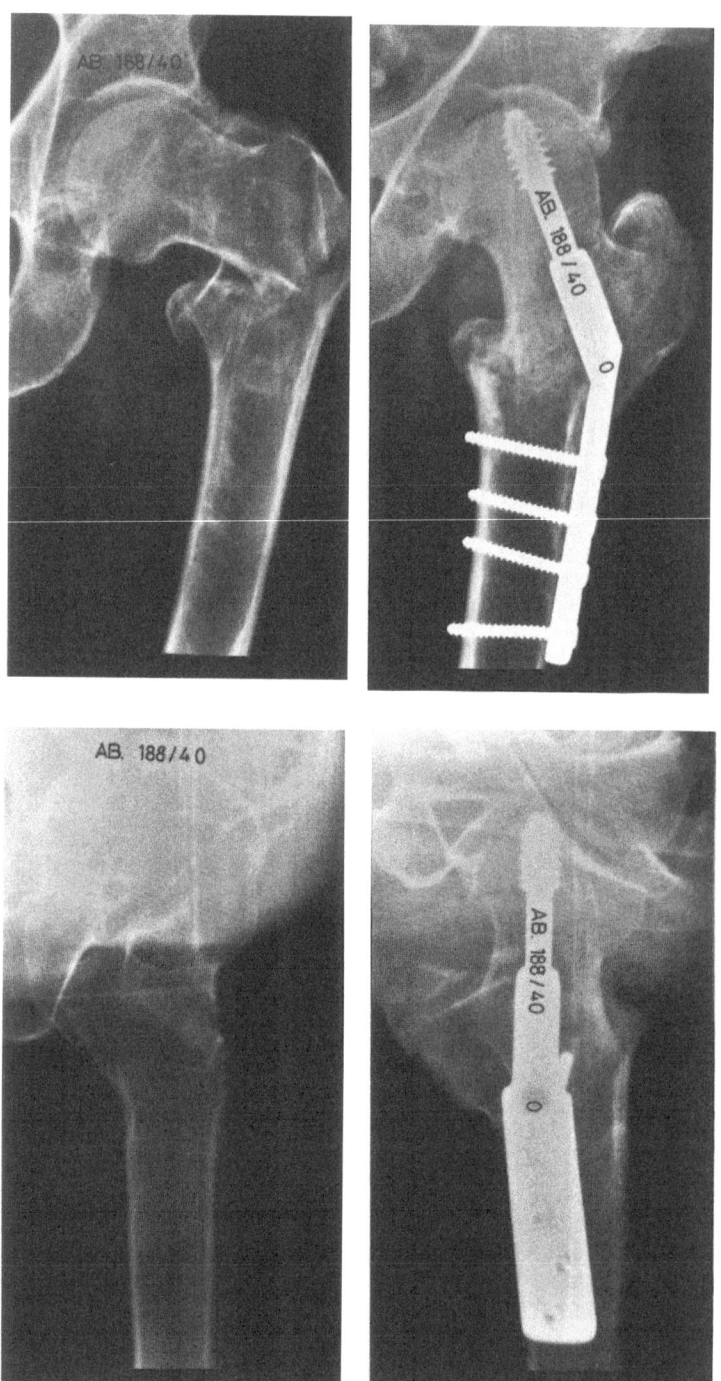

Fig. 37. Type A.2.3 fracture in a 69-year-old woman. 145° DHS, side plate too short in osteoporotic bone; secondary plate stripping. Reoperation with longer side plate and bone cement

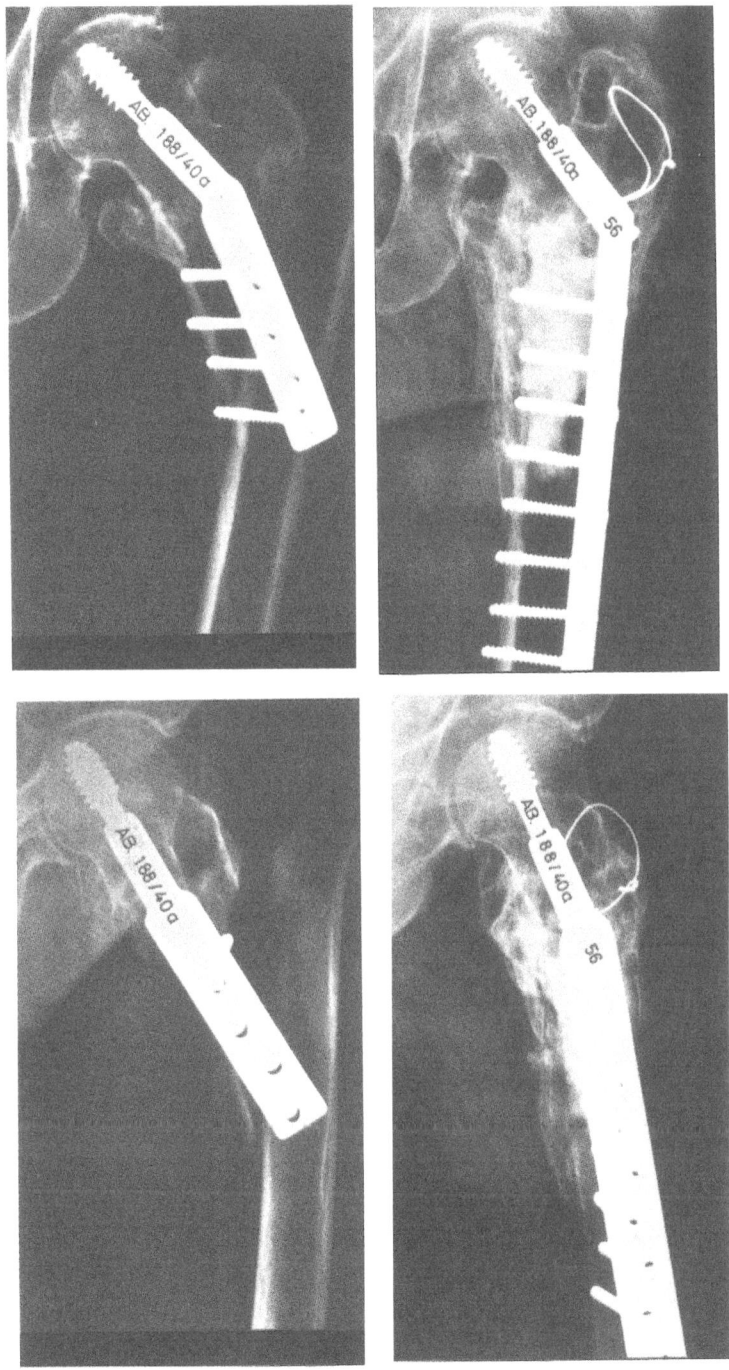

Fig. 37 (continued)

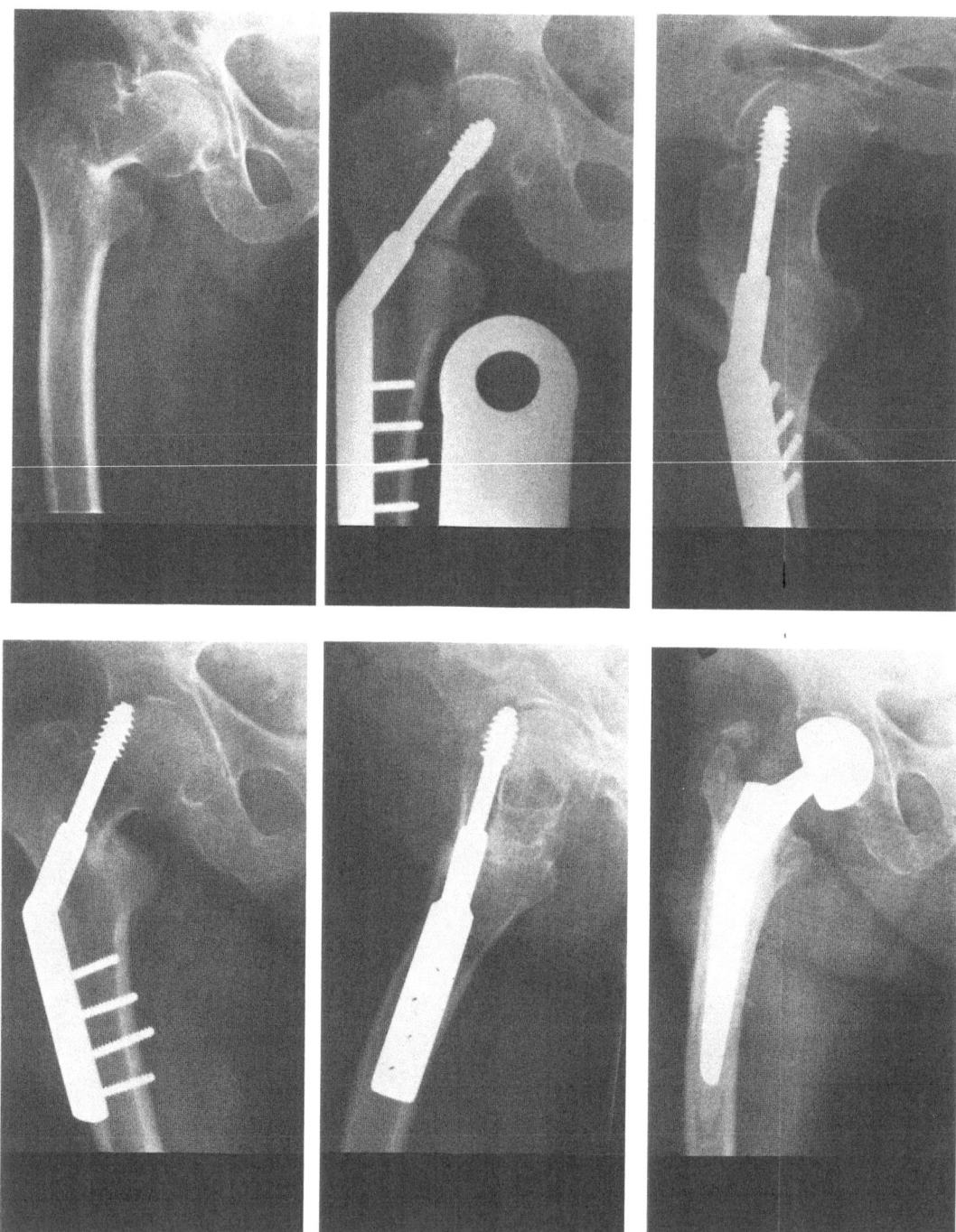

Fig. 38. Woman, 84 years old, with type A.1.2 fracture. Incorrect placement of DHS in the weak anterosuperior quadrant. This is the most frequent technical error. It can be avoided by checking the correct placement of the guide pin with the image intensifier. Subsequent penetration of the lag screw into the hip joint. Removal of the DHS and implantation of an endoprosthesis 2 months later.

In such cases a primary prosthetic replacement must be considered when the bad placement of the DHS is recognized

5 Clinical Results: A Comparison

A great number of different implants have been recommended for the stabilization of trochanteric fractures. As discussed before (Sect. 2), the treatment of stable trochanteric fractures is easy with any implant, but problems are frequent with unstable fracture types. An optimal implant should fulfill the following criteria:

1. The operation should be technically easy. Trochanteric fractures are very frequent, and every surgeon should be able to stabilize these fractures correctly by a short and technically not very demanding procedure.
2. The implant should be suitable, if possible, for all fracture types. Immediate weight bearing should also be possible for unstable fracture types, as we know that elderly patients are not able to bear weight partially.
3. The complication rate should be low (infection and implant complications).

During the past 10 years the authors from Basel have used three different types of implants for trochanteric fractures:

1. Dynamic hip screws ($n = 268$)
2. Angled blade plates ($n = 262$)
3. Ender's nails ($n = 100$)

We have compared the three series according to the criteria mentioned above. A similar number of unstable fracture types in each series is an important prerequisite for such a comparison. Each series had about 50% of unstable cases.

Dynamic Hip Screw

Owing to well-designed instrumentation the procedure is relatively easy. The mean duration of the operation is shorter than that for angled blade plates. One or two image intensifiers are indispensable.

The DHS allows stabilization of all types of trochanteric fractures, including those with a subtrochanteric extension. Postoperative weight bearing is also possible in unstable cases (50.5% of our series).

Infections were far less frequent (2.2%) than in the series with angled blade plates. The frequency of implant complications was also lower with the DHS than with the other two implants (see Table 1).

Table 1. Complications using the DHS for internal fixation (*n* = 268)

	No. (%)	Reoperation
Infection	6 (2.2)	4
Hematoma	5 (1.9)	3
Malrotation of the thigh	5 (1.9)	2
Implant complication	4 (1.5)	2
Avascular necrosis	2 (0.8)	2
Total	22 (8.3)	13 (4.5%)

Angled Blade Plates

Stabilization of trochanteric fractures with the AO/ASIF angled blade plate is a technically demanding procedure. There is no "forgiving" with this system; any small deviation from the recommended technique causes problems.

We have used the angled blade plates for all types of fractures. Immediate postoperative weight bearing was also allowed for the 50% of unstable cases in the series.

Unfortunately, complications are frequent (Table 2): the infection rate of 6% is scarcely acceptable. Even more disappointing is the frequency of implant complications (15%), such as fatigue fracture of the implant, blade penetration into the acetabulum or actual cutout of the blade, and pullout or breakage of screws in the lateral cortex of the femur.

Table 2. Complications using the angled blade plates (*n* = 262)

	No. (%)	Reoperation
Infection	15 (6)	11
Implant complication	44 (15)	32
Avascular necrosis	1 (0.4)	1

Ender's Nails

The Ender procedure [14] is technically easy. The operation is short and blood loss is minimal. A fracture table and an image intensifier are indispensable.

Our limited experience shows that unstable fractures cannot be sufficiently stabilized to allow immediate weight bearing. Excepting a few enthusiastically positive reports, this coincides with the literature [24].

Table 3. Complications using Ender's nails

	Basel series (%) n=100		Böhler (%) n=2137	
		Reoperation		Reoperation
Supracondylar fracture during operation	1		0.2	
Infections: superficial	2	1	1.9	
deep	0	0	0.28	
Implant complications	24	20		
− Penetration of nails into the hip joint	7	7	1.4	1.9
− Distal migration of the nails with varus deformity of the fracture	8	8		
− Distal migration of the nails with severe pain, without varus deformity	9	5	9.9	

The main advantage of this technique is the absence of deep infection.

On the other hand, implant complications (nail penetration into the hip joint, distal migration of the nails with varus deformity of the fracture) are very frequent, if unstable fractures are also mobilized with full weight bearing. Reoperations might also be necessary because of severe pain at the knee, following distal migration of single nails without varus dislocation of the fracture. Malrotation of the thigh (external rotation) is very frequent, even in Böhler's [2] series.

On the basis of this comparative study we are convinced that, at present, the DHS is the optimal implant for trochanteric fractures, including those with subtrochanteric extension [24, 40]. The operation is *technically easy, suitable for all fracture types,* allows early weight bearing, and has an *acceptable complication rate.*

6 Laboratory Tests with the DHS

P. Comte

During the healing period of a trochanteric fracture the implant takes over a part of the load which is transmitted from the hip joint to the femoral shaft. Consequently, the screw-plate device must be constructed to withstand the repeated load which develops during weight bearing. A certain margin of safety has to be taken into account.

To perform the function of a partial weight-bearing appliance the sliding screw-plate implant should meet the following criteria:

- The screw-plate assembly should resist a certain number of repeated bending loads without failure, to permit the fracture to unite.
- The shaft of the screw should be able to slide within the barrel of the plate to allow for impaction at the fracture site.

The purpose of this investigation was to determine the intrinsic mechanical strength of the devices under static and dynamic conditions and to evaluate the factors controlling the sliding of the screw.

Methods and Materials

The mechanical properties of the DHS implant (Synthes type 281.16, 135°) have been determined in bending tests and compared with those of the angled blade plate (Synthes type 238.68, 130°). Load-deflection characteristics and fatigue curves were obtained using a special test fixture shown in Figs. 39 and 40. To avoid the problems created by fixing the nail plate with bone screws a C-fixture with six screws was used (as recommended by ASTM [American Society for Testing of Materials], revision of F 384-73, the Norm for Static Bend Testing of Nail Plates).

The plate was mounted in the test fixture with the barrel pointing in the horizontal position (Fig. 39), while the load component (F) was applied perpendicularly to the shaft of the screw at a distance of 65 mm from the plate-barrel junction; 40 mm of the DHS plate and 27 mm of the angled blade plate (corresponding to one screw hole) stuck out of the plate fixture.

Fatigue tests were performed using the arrangement shown in Fig. 40 (a motor-driven eccentric system applies) a constant bending deformation to the plate. The corresponding force is measured dynamically with a piezoelectric sensor (Kistler type 9021) and a peak amplitude detector allows the maximum applied force to be recorded. To ensure that only vertical forces are transmitted a ball joint is used on the load-transmitting arm. This feature is particularly important

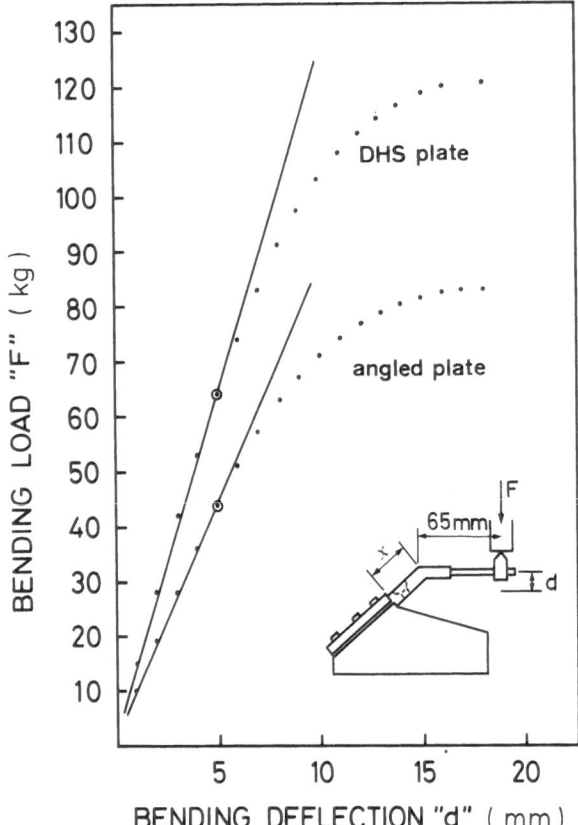

Fig. 39. Load-deflection diagrams and test fixture. *F,* load; *x,* length of plate protruding from plate fixture; *d,* bending deflection

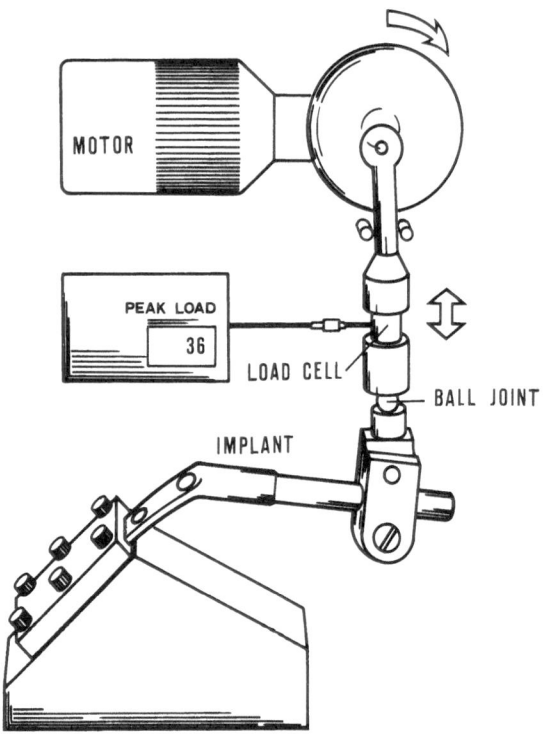

Fig. 40. Test fixture

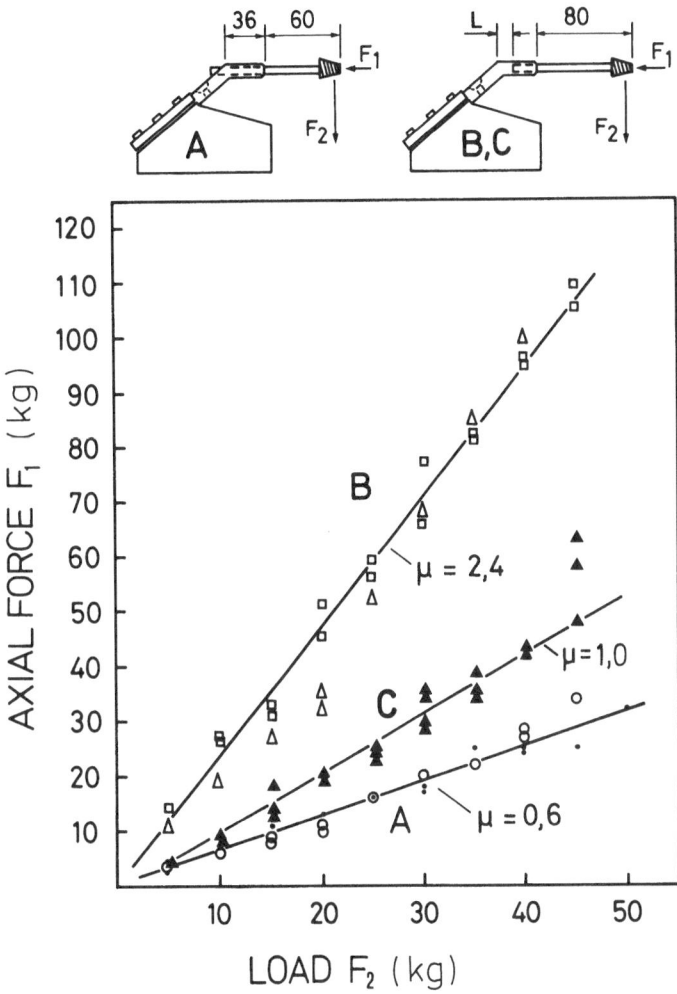

Fig. 41. Fixtures for testing sliding characteristics and corresponding diagrams. Test conditions A, B, C: *A*, screw fully engaged in barrel (*L*=0 mm); *B*, screw half engaged (*L*= 18 mm); *C*, screw partially engaged (*L*=10 mm). *L*, distance from end of lag screw to plate angle (*between opposing arrows*); μ, coefficient of friction

when large bending deflections are applied to the plate. All measurements were done in mode $k = \sigma$ ($k = \sigma$ min/σ max) of unidirectional bending. The fatigue measurements were performed at a frequency of 3 Hz under dry conditions. The telescoping possibility of the device was locked for the DHS test.

In order to determine the sliding characteristics of the screw-plate assembly the set up shown in Fig. 41 was studied. The plate is fixed with the barrel in the horizontal position while a static perpendicular load F_2 is applied at the end of the screw. For a given load F_2 a gradually increasing force F_1 is then applied on the axis of the screw until sliding is initiated. The force F_1 was monitored using a load cell (Kistler piezoelectric sensor type 9021) and calibrated weights of up to 50 kg were used for load F_2. The apparent coefficient of friction μ, defined as the ratio of the axial force F_1 required to initiate sliding to the load F_2, has been determined for different situations. Two factors were presumed

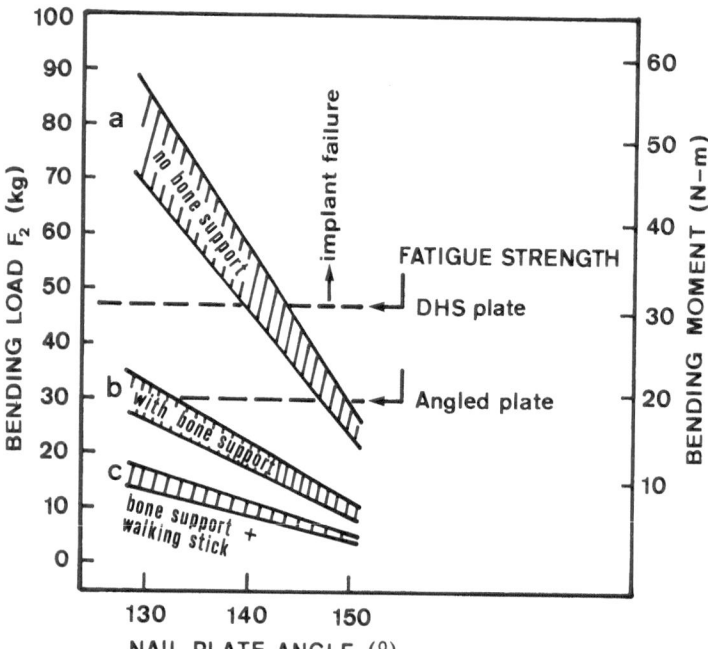

Fig. 42. Influence of plate angle on bending load under varying conditions

for each test: the surface condition of material and the engagement of the distal portion of the screw within the barrel of the plate.

The sliding properties of the screw have been computed for different plate angles for the situation depicted in Fig. 42. The resultant force applied to the screw R in the case where there is no bone support can be resolved into components parallel ($F_1 = R \cos \alpha$) and perpendicular ($F_2 = R \sin \alpha$) to the screw axis. The force F_2 is responsible for creating a bending moment in the screw and a resistive frictional force given by the product μF_2. When the parallel force F_1 exceeds the maximum static frictional force μF_2, sliding can be initiated ($F_1/\mu F_2 > 1$).

Assuming that forces on the hip are applied at an angle of 70° to the horizontal plane [21, 37, 41], the ratio of the available to the resistive force can be obtained as a function of the plate angle β, and is given by the following expression:

$$\frac{F_1}{\mu F_2} = \frac{1}{\mu \tan 160° - \beta}.$$

The coefficients of friction (Fig. 41) are then introduced in this formula and the ratio $F_1/\mu F_2$ is calculated for the different plate angles. The coefficient of friction is defined as the ratio of the force parallel to the screw barrel F_1 that is required to initiate sliding with the force applied perpendicularly to the barrel F_2 (Fig. 41).

The materials used in this study were original stainless steel AO/ASIF implants whose properties are described in Table 4. Their metallurgical properties and suitability as implant material have been described elsewhere [9, 38, 45].

Table 4. Characteristics of implants

AO/ASIF stainless steel	Type	Plate dimensions (mm)	Bending[a]			
			Yield strength (N-m)	Ultimate strength (N-m)	Rigidity (N-m²)	Fatigue strength (N-m)
Dynamic hip screw, DHS	281.16, 135°	6 × 19	57	107	30	28
Angled plate	238.68, 130°	6 × 16	35	66	16	18

[a] Bending properties obtained from Figs. 39 and 43. The shaft of the femur has a breaking strength of 250 N-m and a bending rigidity of 310 N-m² [47]; the force required to produce experimental fractures of the femur head varies from 300 to 800 kg [16]

Results and Discussion

Mechanical Strength of Hip Plates

Figure 39 represents the load-deflection characteristic of the implants. Under the test conditions previously described (lever arm of 65 mm), the DHS plate has an elastic limit of 65 kg (corresponding bending yield strength of 57 N-m) compared with 45 kg (yield strength of 35 N-m) for the angled blade plate. These values indicate the load, after elimination of which no permanent deformation (plastic deformation) of the plate will result.

For both plates the elastic limit corresponds to a bending deflection of 5 mm. The ultimate bending strength is also significantly higher for the DHS plate. The strength superiority of the DHS implant is due mainly to its increased cross-sectional area; its bending rigidity, however, is about two times that of the angled plate (see Table 4).

Figure 43 represents the fatigue curves of the implants for loads up to 160 kg. Each square or triangle indicates the number of cycles necessary to initiate cracking. Since the test machine applies a constant deformation to the implant, cracking is detected by a sudden fall in the recorded load, as illustrated in Fig. 44. The load limit at which no failure occurs, called the "fatigue strength", can be estimated from Fig. 43. For the DHS plate a value of 28 N-m (corresponding to 47 kg of applied load) was measured, compared with 18 N-m (30 kg) for the angled blade plate. In the low-cycle range (10^4–10^5) the DHS plate is capable of withstanding much higher loads (up to 150 kg) than the angled blade plate is (limited to 90 kg). For an identical load level the DHS plate tolerates three times more fatigue cycles.

The purpose of this study was to determine the mechanical properties of the implants under load. In order to measure performance during physiological loading, other factors would have to be introduced to evaluate what could possibly bring the implant to fail.

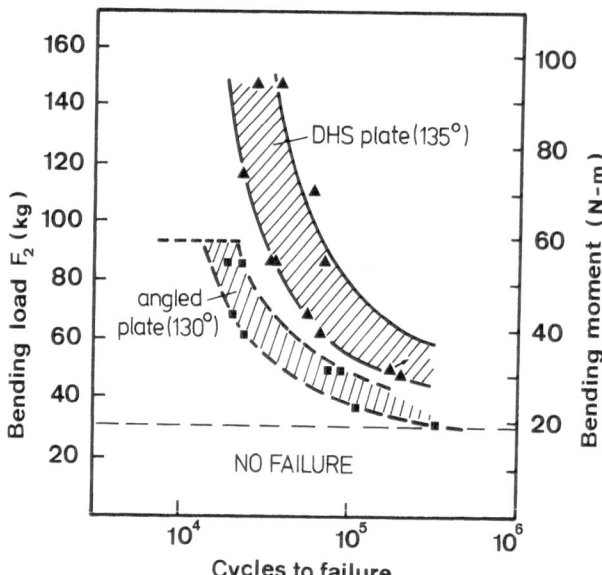

Fig. 43. Fatigue curves for DHS and angled plate

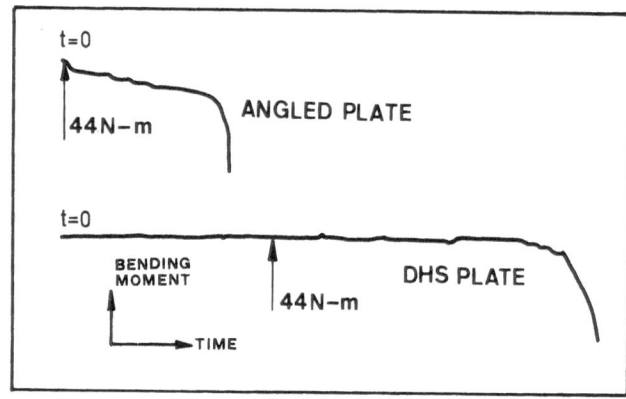

Fig. 44. Fatigue curves. Cracking of the implant is detected by sudden fall in recorded load. Cracking occurs earlier with the angled blade plate

Studies by Kilvington and Goodman, Paul, Pauwels, and Rydell [27, 36, 37, 41] demonstrate that the forces about the hip are highest during the single-limb stand phase and that they represent 1.8–2.3 times body weight. From the situation shown in Fig. 45, the force F_2 is responsible for creating the bending moment and is calculated as a function of the plate angle as follows:

$$F_2 = R \sin \alpha = (1.8-2.3) \text{ body wt} \sin (160° - \beta).$$

Assuming the weight of 75 kg for an average patient, F_2 is represented in Fig. 42 for three different situations: (a) with no bony support the load is entirely transmitted to the implant; (b) in a stable fracture (good bony support) 50%–75% of the total load can be absorbed by the bone [16, 17, 43]; (c) if, in addition, a walking stick is used on the uninjured side, the weight bearing should be reduced by half [1].

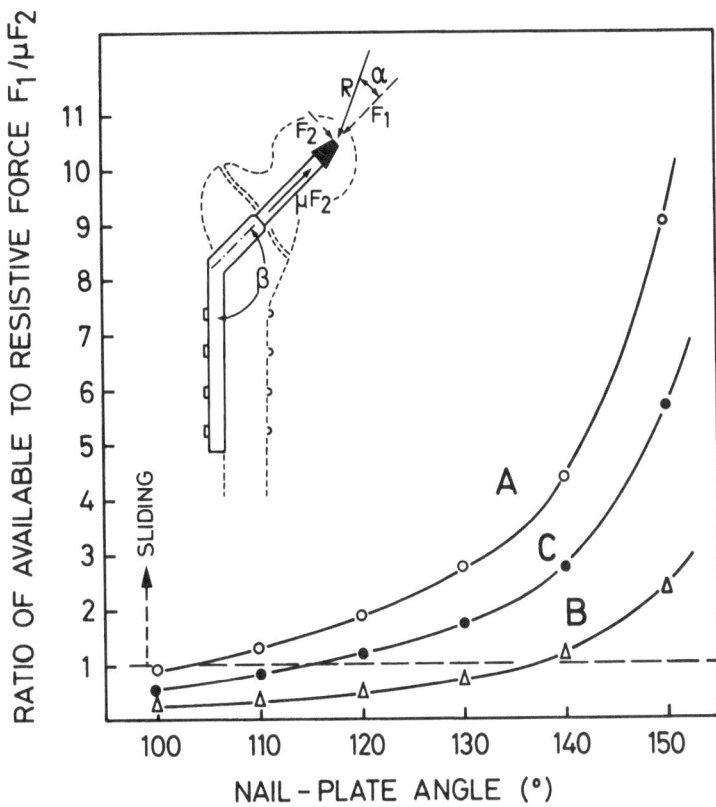

Fig. 45. Sliding characteristics under varying conditions. *A, B, C,* test conditions (cf. Fig. 41); *R,* resultant of F_1 and F_2 (cf. Fig. 41); α, angle between resultant and axial force; β, plate angle; μ, coefficient of friction

In Fig. 42 the fatigue strength of the DHS and angled blade plate has also been indicated. It may also be seen from Fig. 42 that with the use of an angled blade plate with angles of 140°–150°, the bending load applied to the implant is appreciably reduced compared with plates with smaller angles (130°–135°), especially in completely unstable situations (a above) where the bending load exceeds the fatigue strength of the angled blade plates. The estimated safety factors offered by the DHS plate in the cases of stable fixation are 1.5 and 3.6 for the 135° and 150° plates respectively. These results also suggest that more care must be taken when using angled blade plates. In order to obtain a sufficient safety margin for the implant (angled blade plate) only partial weight bearing may be tolerated. With 50% weight bearing (situation c above) a fatigue failure of the angled blade plate can be avoided. In vivo measurements of bending moments of hip nails confirm the data presented in Fig. 42 [4]. During unassisted walking the hip nails were submitted to peak bending moments of 20 N-m.

It must be emphasized, however, that hip screw implants can withstand early full weight bearing only if adequate reduction of the fracture has been obtained or if a new bony support has been found by "telescoping" of the screw within the barrel.

Sliding Characteristics of the Screw

These experiments were done to determine the forces that will initiate sliding in relation to conditions such as the engagement of the screw within the barrel, the nail-plate angle, and the surface condition of the implant material.

In Fig. 41 forces F_1 have been measured for loads F_2 ranging from 5 to 50 kg in three different situations:

A – The screw is fully engaged in the barrel ($L=0$ mm). In this situation the forces to initiate sliding are the lowest. The coefficient of friction calculated from the straight line is $\mu=0.6$ and the highest force recorded was 30 kg.

B – The screw is half engaged in the barrel ($L=18$ mm). The sliding forces in this case are the highest with a correspondingly high coefficient of friction. Sliding forces of up to 110 kg (for a 50-kg load) have been detected.

C – The screw is not completely engaged in the barrel ($L=10$ mm). In this case a coefficient of friction $\mu=1.0$ has been determined.

From the data presented in Fig. 41 it can be seen that the coefficient of friction remains constant in the range 5–50 kg applied load.

Figure 45 illustrates two properties of the sliding system. First, it indicates the critical angle of the nail-plate junction below which no sliding will occur. Second, the factor $F_1/\mu F_2$ provides a measure of the force available for bone impaction. In the situations A and C ($L=0$ mm and $L=10$ mm; see Fig. 41) sliding will occur even at the low angle of 135°. In the optimal situation C, the force available for impaction will be two times the resistive force for the 135° DHS plate and about six times the resistive force for the 150° DHS plate. When the screw is only half engaged in the barrel, jamming of the shaft of the screw in the barrel is observed for the 135° plate but not for the 150° DHS. Similar observations have been made by Kyle et al. [29] on various other compression hip screw devices. The potential for jamming, which can lead to complications such as loss of reduction or failure due to fatigue, is decreased by maximum engagement of the screw in the barrel and by the use of a plate with a high angle.

We are well aware of the limitations of our measurements performed under dry conditions. However, the same experiments repeated on hip screws retrieved from patients gave the same results. Only very slight increases in the coefficient of friction were observed. Moreover, the good uniformity in the reproducibility of the coefficient of friction μ tends to demonstrate that this parameter is a constant material property.

Conclusions

Static and dynamic load testing and determination of sliding properties of screw-plate hip implants were performed, and parameters such as the angle of the plate and the length of the engagement of the screw within the barrel were considered.

In comparison with the results obtained for the angled blade plate, the DHS plate has a higher yield strength ($+63\%$) and superior fatigue strength ($+56\%$). Dynamic bending loads of up to 150 kg have been applied 20000 times without failure. When bony support is provided, the plate is submitted to stresses that will not usually lead to implant failure. The DHS implant is capable of sustaining the total weight of patients even with unstable fractures, but only for a limited number of cycles.

The static conditions governing the sliding of the screw were determined. For plates with low angles (130°) it is important that the screw has a maximum engagement in the barrel to avoid jamming. Plates with high angles (150°) may be implanted with the screw only half engaging the barrel without risk of jamming, but the risk of disengagement of the screw plate [3, 6] must then be considered. Plates with a high angle are subjected to lower bending loads and the force necessary for bone impaction is also lower. The question of which kind of DHS plate – high- or low-angle – should be used is still controversial. Low-angle screw plates are usually preferred owing to their ease of insertion. The present study confirms that they may be used quite safely.

7 Summary

Sliding compression screws are – at present – the optimal implants for trochanteric and selected femoral neck and subtrochanteric fractures [12, 13, 23, 24, 28, 35, 40]. The surgical procedure is relatively easy, the results are good, and the complication rate is acceptable.

Although screw plates with high angles (145°–150°) have certain biomechanical advantages, the 135° DHS plate is preferred owing to the ease of insertion.

8 References

1. Blount W (1956) Don't throw away the cane. J Bone Joint Surg 38-A:695
2. Böhler N, Kuderna H (1977) Ergebnisse der Endernagelung in Österreich unter spezieller Berücksichtigung der Fälle des Lorenz-Böhler-Krankenhauses. Arch Orthop Unfallchir 88:339–346
3. Brodell JD, Leve AR (1983) Disengagement and intrapelvic protrusion of the screw from a sliding screw-plate device. J Bone Joint Surg 65-A:697
4. Brown RH, Burstein AH, Frankel VH (1982) Telemetering in vivo loads from nail-plate implants. J Biomech 15:815
5. Burnett JW, Gustilo RB, Williams DN, Kind AC (1980) Prophylactic antibiotics in hip fractures. A double-blind, prospective study. J Bone Joint Surg 62-A:457
6. Cameron HU, Graham JD (1980) Retention of the compression screw in sliding screw-plate devices. Clin Orthop 146:219
7. Clawson DK (1957) Intertrochanteric fracture of the hip. Am J Surg 93:580
8. Clawson D (1964) Trochanteric fractures treated by the sliding screw plate fixation method. J Trauma 4:737
9. Comte P (1984) Metallurgical observations of biomaterials. In: Boretos J, Murray E (eds) Introduction of biomaterials to clinical care, chap. 7. Noyes, Park Ridge (in press)
10. Dimon J, Hughston J (1967) Unstable intertrochanteric fractures of the hip. J Bone Joint Surg 49-A:440
11. Doherty JH, Lyden JP (1979) Intertrochanteric fractures of the hip treated with the hip compression screw. Clin Orthop 141:184
12. Doppelt S (1980) The sliding compression screw – today's best answer for stabilization of intertrochanteric hip fractures. Orthop Clin North Am 11:507
13. Ecker ML, Joyce JJ III, Kohl EJ (1975) The treatment of trochanteric hip fractures using a compression screw. J Bone Joint Surg 57-A:23
14. Ender HG (1976) Richtlinien zur Behandlung per- und subtrochanterer Brüche mit Federnägeln. Aktuel Traumatol 6:155
15. Evans EM (1949) The treatment of trochanteric fractures of the femur. J Bone Joint Surg 31-B:190
16. Frankel VH (1969) Mechanical principles for internal fixation of the femoral head. Acta Orthop Scand 117:427
17. Frankel VH (1960) The femoral neck, fracture mechanism and internal fixation – an experimental study. Charles and Thomas, Springfield, Ill
18. Ganz R (1981) Die trochanteren Femurfrakturen. Habilitationsschrift, University of Bern
19. Ganz R, Thomas RJ, Hammerle CP (1979) Trochanteric fractures of the femur. Treatment and results. Clin Orthop 138:30
20. Harrington KD, Johnson JO (1973) Management of comminuted unstable intertrochanteric fractures. J Bone Joint Surg 55-A:1367
21. Inman VT (1947) Functional aspects of the abductor muscles of the hip. J Bone Joint Surg 29:461
22. Iversen HG (1965) Medial femoral neck fractures treated with Pohl's sliding screw. Acta Chir Scand 129:477

23. Jacobs RR, McClain O, Armstrong HJ (1980) Internal fixation of intertrochanteric hip fractures: a clinical and biomechanical study. Clin Orthop 146:62
24. Jensen JS, Sonne-Holm S, Tøndevold E (1980) Unstable trochanteric fractures, a comparative analysis of four methods of internal fixation. Acta Orthop Scand 51:949
25. Jensen JS, Tøndevold E, Sonne-Holm S (1980) Stable trochanteric fractures, a comparative analysis of four methods of internal fixation. Acta Orthop Scand 51:811
26. Kempf JH, Jaeger J, Freund D, Renault S, Bitar S, Konsbruck R, Butel J, Faure C, Bonnel F (1981) Aspects mécaniques de l'osteosynthèse des fractures du col du fémur. Etude comparative des différents moyens d'osteosynthèse. Rev Chir Orthop 67:59
27. Kilvington M, Goodman RMF (1981) In vivo hip joint forces recorded on a strain-gauged "English" prosthesis using an implanted transmitter. Eng Med 10:176–187
28. Kyle RF, Gustilo RB, Premer RF (1979) Analysis of 622 intertrochanteric hip fractures. J Bone Joint Surg 61-A:216
29. Kyle RF, Wright TM, Burstein AH (1980) Biomechanical analysis of the sliding characteristics of compression hip screws. J Bone Joint Surg 62-A:1308
30. Laskin RS, Gruber MA, Zimmerman AJ (1979) Intertrochanteric fractures of the hip in the elderly: a retrospective analysis of 236 cases. Clin Orthop 141:188
31. Massie WK (1956) Functional fixation of intracapsular fractures of the hip. Proc Am Acad Orthop Surg
32. Massie WK (1958) Functional fixation of femoral neck fractures with telescoping nail technique. Clin Orthop 12:230
33. Müller ME, Nazarian S (1981) Classification et documentation AO des fractures du fémur. Rev Chir Orthop 67:297
34. Müller ME, Allgöwer M, Willenegger H, Schneider R (1979) Manual of internal fixation. Springer, Berlin Heidelberg New York
35. Mulholland RC, Gunn DR (1972) Sliding screw plate fixation of intertrochanteric fractures. J Trauma 12:581
36. Paul JP (1976) Force actions transmitted by joints in the human body. Proc R Soc Lond [Biol] 192:163
37. Pauwels F (1935) Der Schenkelhalsbruch – ein mechanisches Problem. Enke, Stuttgart
38. Pohler O, Straumann F (1975) Characteristics of the stainless steel ASIF/AO implants. AO Bulletin, September
39. Pugh WL (1955) A self-adjusting nail plate for fracture about the hip joint. J Bone Joint Surg 37A:1085
40. Regazzoni P, Jaeger G, Op den Winkel R, Isay M, Allgöwer M (1981) Ein Vergleich verschiedener Implantate bei pertrochanteren Femurfrakturen. Helv Chir Acta 48:677
41. Rydell NW (1966) Forces acting on the femoral head prosthesis. Acta Orthop Scand [Suppl N 86] 93:71
42. Sahlstrand T (1974) The Richards compression and sliding hip-screw system in the treatment of intertrochanteric fractures. Acta Orthop Scand 45:213
43. Sarmiento A (1963) Intertrochanteric fracture of the femur. 150°-angle nail fixation and early rehabilitation: a preliminary report of 100 cases. J Bone Joint Surg 45-A:706
44. Schumpelick W, Jantzen PM (1955) A new principle in the operative treatment of trochanteric fractures of the femur. J Bone Joint Surg 37-A:693
45. Steinemann S (1980) Corrosion of surgical implants. In: Winter GD, Leray JL, de Groot D (eds) Evaluation of biomaterials. Wiley, Chichester, pp 1–34
46. Waddell JP (1979) Subtrochanteric fractures of the femur: a review of 130 patients. J Trauma 19:582
47. Yamada H (1970) Strength of biological materials: mechanical properties of locomotor organs and tissues. Williams and Wilkins, Baltimore, pp 19–105

9 Subject Index

R.Bombelli

Osteoarthritis of the Hip

Classification and Pathogenesis
The Role of Osteotomy as a Consequent Therapy

With a Foreword by M.E.Müller
2nd, revised and enlarged edition. 1983. 374 figures (partly in colour).
XVIII, 386 pages. ISBN 3-540-11422-X

Renato Bombelli, Professor of Orthopedics at the University of Milan, has
treated more than 1500 cases of primary and secondary osteoarthritis of the
hip in the last 20 years. This book is the result of his clinical, radiological and
surgical observations in the course of this distinguished career. In it, Prof.
Bombelli details the biomechanics of the normal and diseased hip and
shows that the natural healing process can be accelerated through changes
induced by surgery on the forces acting on the hip. Bombelli's intertrochanteric osteotomy subjects the superior capsule of the hip to tension to induce
osteophyte formation along the superior lip of the acetabulum, forming a
physiological "shelf" and thereby increasing the weight bearing area of the
hip. His procedure is shown to produce excellent results, particularly in
young adults. For this second, revised and enlarged edition, Prof. Bombelli
has further refined his classification of osteoarthritis of the hip, his theory of
hip biomechanics, and the indications for osteotomy. He has also included
updated clinical statistics which lend credence to his conclusion that,
whereas the best hip replacement is of unknown but certainly finite duration, a hip healed after osteotomy will often last a lifetime.

The Cementless Fixation of Hip Endoprostheses

Editor: **E.Morscher**

1984. 230 figures. XV, 284 pages. ISBN 3-540-12254-0

This book examines the problems associated with hip endoprostheses,
emphasizing the possibilities and limitations of cementless fixation.
It surveys the biomechanics of prosthetic loosening, the biochemistry of
implants, and the choice of implant material. Special consideration is also
given to the design of acetabular prostheses, the character of the prosthetic
surface, and the elastic and mechanical properties of the implant.
The volume comprises the papers presented at a symposium on cementless
hip endoprostheses, held in Basle in June, 1982. This was the first symposium ever held which dealt exclusively with this topic. There were presen-
tations on various methods of hip endoprosthetic attachment used at
present, as well as those still being tested and assessed. This is the first
comprehensive account of cementless hip prostheses and provides an over-
view of the special problems in this field. It summarizes the current state of
knowledge and indicates the direction of future developments.

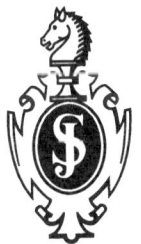

Springer-Verlag
Berlin
Heidelberg
New York
Tokyo

P.G.J.Maquet

Biomechanics of the Hip

As Applied to Osteoarthritis and Related Conditions
1984. Approx. 285 figures. Approx. 56 tables. Approx. 300 pages
ISBN 3-540-13257-0

Surgery of the Hip Joint

Volume 1
Editor: R.G.Tronzo
2nd edition. 1984. Approx. 500 figures. Approx. 548 pages
ISBN 3-540-90922-2

The Intertrochanteric Osteotomy

Editor: J.Schatzker
1984. Approx. 101 figures, approx. 18 tables. Approx. 300 pages
ISBN 3-540-10719-3

E.W.Somerville

Displacement of the Hip in Childhood

Aetiology, Management and Sequelae
1982. 262 figures. XIII, 200 pages. ISBN 3-540-10936-6

J.Charnley

Low Friction Arthroplasty of the Hip

Theory and Practice
1979. 440 figures, 205 in colour, 22 tables. X, 376 pages
ISBN 3-540-08893-8

R.Liechti

Hip Arthrodesis and Associated Problems

Foreword by M.E.Müller, B.G.Weber
Translated from the German edition by P.A.Casey
1978. 266 figures, 35 tables. XII, 269 pages. ISBN 3-540-08614-5

F.Pauwels

Biomechanics of the Normal and Diseased Hip

Theoretical Foundation, Technique and Results of Treatment
An Atlas
Translated from the German by R.J.Furlong, P.Maquet
1976. 305 figures (in 853 separate illustrations). VIII, 276 pages
ISBN 3-540-07428-7

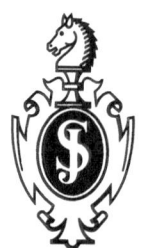

Springer-Verlag
Berlin
Heidelberg
New York
Tokyo